THE MAGIC OF THE MINIMUM DOSE

By the same author
MORE MAGIC OF THE MINIMUM DOSE
HOMOEOPATHY FOR THE FIRST-AIDER
HOMOEOPATHY IN EPIDEMIC DISEASES
A PHYSICIAN'S POSY

THE MAGIC OF THE
MINIMUM DOSE

EXPERIENCES AND CASES

BY
DR. DOROTHY SHEPHERD

Health Science Press
The C.W. Daniel Company Ltd.
1 Church Path, Saffron Walden, Essex, England

First published 1938
Second (revised) Edition 1946
Third Edition 1964
Second Impression November 1973
Third Impression January 1979
Fourth Impression February 1985

ISBN 0 85032 112 3

Printed in Great Britain by
The Eastern Press Limited
London and Reading

CONTENTS

FOREWORD

ONE feels that Homœopathy is not clearly understood; it has been the Cinderella of Medicine for so long; it is time that this lowly hand-maiden should shed her cloak of humility and come out of her obscurity and boldly proclaim what good she can do. This account of some experiences in the daily harassing life of a humble homœopathic disciple is given in order to spread the knowledge of Homœopathy; not as a self advertisement. God forbid! There are hundreds more in the British Isles and in America and on the continent of Europe who could do the teaching of Homœopathy and tell of this miraculous power of the homœopathic drug in sickness—so much better.

Some of the following pages appeared in *Heal Thyself* (*The Homœopathic World*), and by request of the Publisher have been revised, with additions. If, after reading them, some would be led into studying Homœopathy for themselves or to ask their doctors to interest themselves in Homœopathy, one would be content.

This is not meant to be a textbook of Homœopathy or a complete book on clinical homœopathic therapeutics. They are just experiences picked out at random to illustrate the mighty truths that are hidden in Homœopathy, and to show the sometimes wonderful results which can be obtained, if the directions given by the masters are followed. There are no exaggerations in the reports of the cases mentioned: they are plain unvarnished truths of incidents that actually happened.

May Homœopathy flourish and grow from strength to strength!

DOROTHY SHEPHERD

FOREWORD TO THE 2ND EDITION

MY publisher tells me that a 2nd edition is called for. Naturally it is gratifying to hear that this child of my brain was not still born and has been appreciated. Now this reprint gives me a chance to explain my title "The Magic of the Minimum Dose" which was chosen purposely, not for its attractive alliteration alone, but for its hidden significance. The word "magic" in the course of years has changed its original meaning and degenerated so that it now implies sorcery and witchcraft.

Etymologically the name magic was derived through the Greeks from the Zend (one of the original root languages of the ancient East) where Mag or Magh stood for sage or priest. The Chaldeans, another ancient people, altered the word to Maghdrin, which corresponds to secret philosophy or high wisdom.

The ancient Magi combined the offices of priest, astronomer, scientist and architect; it is they who built those gigantic temples, long ages ago, whose mighty ruins, the only remnants of a forgotten civilization, were found in Arabia after the Great War of 1914-18, by a travelling American who brought wonderful photographs of these basalt and marble temples and palaces which leave us struck dumb with amazement.

Yes, those magi did not only know the physical laws applying to architecture, to medicine and astronomy, but many other laws of the supernatural forces going beyond the three dimensions, the knowledge of which we have lost completely. What forces did they employ in building the pyramids; what is the secret of the Sphinx? We do not know in spite of all our so-called progress.

And you recall the three wise men or magi of the New Testament, who while studying the high firmament of the heavens, were led by their inner knowledge to follow the "Star" to the little town of Bethlehem, there to fall down and worship the Christ Child, the prophesied Saviour of the world.

Yes, I chose the title "Magic" with deliberate intent; it stands for the High Wisdom of the power and the forces hidden in the infinitesimal minimum doses which are the spirit of the medicinal substances and agents; it has been described and explained, I trust, in the simplest of words, so that he who will can read and understand.

DOROTHY SHEPHERD

FOREWORD TO THE 3RD EDITION

I LIVED and worked with Dr. Dorothy Shepherd for many years, and came to know and respect her wide knowledge and understanding of Homœopathy, especially in relation to long-standing disease.

Her generosity was boundless in the matter of her personal care and skill for sufferers, and also in her willingness to share her knowledge of Homœopathy with anyone who was willing and anxious to learn of the Art and Science to which she devoted her life. She would teach the lay people with the same care and patience as the medical student—thereby endearing herself to some and antagonising many of her own brethren.

Her driving thought was to bring Homœopathy into the lives of the people, who she realized—as we all do today—were becoming more and more dissatisfied with modern drug treatments. She made endless notes and jottings of thoughts about healing and medicine; information about remedies and accounts of her experiences in clinical practice were scribbled on odd sheets of paper whenever she had a spare moment, wherever she happened to be.

After her sudden passing in 1952, it fell to me to collect these notes together. A busy life with a big homœopathic practice has not left very much time to decipher the pencil jottings and sort into a comprehensible order, but at last this has been done and it will now be possible to publish uniformly with this 3rd edition, further books from Dr. Dorothy Shepherd's great treasury of knowledge and experience.

It is for all who seek the true healing of man's whole being, body, mind and soul, to learn of the Art and Science of a therapy that is based on a firm foundation of proven remedies, and administered according to laws that have been also proven by practical experience and application on healthy men and women—not on the suffering of the animal kingdom through experiment and vivisection.

GWENETH E. ROBINSON
Northam, N. Devon

MY CONVERSION TO HOMŒOPATHIC HIGH POTENCIES

A Personal Experience

FROM my childhood days I have been a Homœopath; in fact I should not have been here at all if it had not been for Homœopathy. For my mother cured herself with homœopathic pilules from a sharp attack of confluent smallpox when the orthodox medical practitioner had given her up, and I was born within a week or two of her recovery. As a member of a homœopathic family, luckily for me, I escaped all the horror of nursery medicines, such as castor oil or Gregory's powders.

The ideals of Homœopathy were rather blurred while I was a medical student. With the foolish superiority of newly acquired knowledge I despised the tiny little globules, which I thought might be good enough for children and their simple ailments. One day I had rather an eye-opener. A bee disliked me and I got a nasty sting on my hand. It swelled, and the inflammation spread up my arm. My mother humbly suggested *Apis* to me. The pain was so great that I took it in desperation and lo and behold! in a few minutes verily all pain and swelling had disappeared. Then I remembered how the previous summer I had been stung on my lip, and how I had been plagued and humiliated and frightened by one-half my face swelling enormously, and the local doctor's remedies had not made the slightest difference for three days. That was orthodox medicine for you! "If only I knew where to learn more about Homœopathy!"

I qualified, and for several years worked strenuously as House Surgeon in various general hospitals, and one day I heard about a School of Homœopathy in Chicago. I thereupon took a busman's holiday and went off to the States in the late autumn. What a voyage that was! Stormy and cold and rainy! I was cooped up in a small cabin with a young mother, and her baby was screaming day and night from teething pains.

I arrived tired and worn in New York and immediately fell a

victim to a feverish chill, due to the effects of a cold northerly wind on a tired-out system. There was I all alone in a foreign country, laid up in a big hotel with a high temperature. What was to be done? Dim recollections from my childhood days came to me. "What were the medicines used? Oh, yes, I have it!" *Aconite* and *Bryonia* 3*x* alternately were taken and in a few hours they reduced my temperature. But I was left with a nasty sequel, a violent frontal sinusitis, an inflammation of the cavities in the bony skull, which caused agonizing pains in my forehead and the bridge of my nose, absolutely blinding in character.

My one idea was to get to Chicago as quickly as possible and get treatment. I have very little recollection of the journey between New York and Chicago, even though I stopped a night at Niagara to see the world-famous Falls. I tried mental treatment of all sorts to ease my head, but nothing was any use. If anything, it got worse and worse. The moment I arrived in Chicago I rushed off to see one of the homœopathic physicians. He was rather brusque and short with me, especially when I told him in my opinion high potencies could not possibly do any good. 2*x* or 3*x* potencies I would grant him, but anything higher —mere moonshine.

He gave me *Nux vomica* on my symptoms, which were, shortly, chill caused by dry cold wind, feeling of icy coldness all through body, could not get warm—even sitting in front of a radiator; shivering as soon as movement started, violent throbbing pain in forehead and nose, worse stooping, worse bending forward, worse warm room, headache worse slightest pressure, generally worse mornings, and withal there was extreme irritability, snappiness and bad temper. I was told: "Take the *Nux vomica* at night but, mind you, it might make you feel worse, a great deal worse, at first. I shall give you one dose of the 100,000th potency." I smiled unbelievingly: I was no fool, I thought the high dilution could have no effect. I might just as well take plain sugar.

Well, I was desperate, I didn't want an operation, which was the only other alternative for the pus in my frontal sinuses. So in the evening I swallowed my *cm.* powder. A very short time afterwards my head felt as if there was a forge inside, such a violent hammering and throbbing and heat—it was like hell let loose. I thought every minute I was going to die with the agony of the pain and prayed for deliverance, when suddenly after half an hour, or maybe an hour, there was blessed relief. The pain left me as suddenly as it had started. I slept all night long. In the morning I got up and tried to stoop and bend forward, which I had been unable to do for several days, and I was free from all discomfort. I sang "Hallelujah, Hallelujah." Twenty-four hours later I took another dose of *Nux cm.* as there was a slight return of the headache and also some difficulty in stooping. I hesitated for fear of starting another aggravation; but this time there was relief at once and no increase of pain at all.

I had learnt two things at one go. First, that high potencies work rapidly and efficaciously, and secondly, that they can cause acute pain and aggravation and should be used with great care. Two valuable lessons indeed. From that day to this I have had no return of frontal sinusitis and, indeed, *Nux vomica* has been a stand-by and valuable help in other cases of acute sinus trouble after colds and nasal catarrhs, both in low potencies (1*x*) and high potencies, whenever indicated.

To continue the story of my conversion to the use of high potencies. I was cured of my acute frontal sinus, but I found I still had a dull heavy feeling all over my head and I could not apply myself at all to any useful work. I could not read for any length of time, I could not remember what I read even; and this heavy stupid feeling was always worse between 10 in the morning and 3 in the afternoon. What particularly worried me was my bad memory, due to not having had a holiday for several years and much over-study. One of my fellow students in Chicago offered to cure me of my cerebral anæmia, and I was only too glad. She advised me to take *Tuberculinum* 1,000th potency, to be repeated in weekly doses. I think I took the 1,000th potency, three doses. Anyway the result again was not far from miraculous. I could read without effort, without being plagued by headaches and, what was better, I could remember what I had read. In fact afterwards, having read a page once or twice over, I could repeat it word by word by heart, an achievement I had not been able to accomplish for several years. Again, a high potency had worked wonders. Are you surprised I tried high potencies on other people? I find that high potencies go deeper and act longer; that is, they act for longer periods and they powerfully stir up the constitution and make a vital difference in the character, temperament and mental make-up of the respective patients.

But a word of warning is not out of place here. Let me impress upon lay people that "high potencies" are not for them to play with. A knowledge of metaphysics, mental philosophy and logic, is necessary before one can hope even humbly to understand their action from a distance. I have been horrified at some people who after reading a book or two on Materia Medica, while they are still in a state of mental indigestion, start to throw their weight about and begin to treat their friends and acquaintances with repeated doses of high potencies, frequently changing the remedies every few days; in their foolish ignorance and vainglory they do more harm to the cause of homœopathy than if they kept to the ordinary run of household remedies.

Let each man stick to his own lasts; the study of medicine and still more the study of homœopathy is a whole-time and life-long occupation.

There are many others, I am fully aware, who having grasped the inner meaning of homœopathy are competent to deal with many of the ailments which beset us on our path through this world of sorrow, without having passed through college and hospital and without possessing a medical qualification. But high potencies although on the other end of the scale are far removed from the material toxic doses, can kill just as surely as poisonous doses of opium, strychnine, etc. High potencies are Vibrations of the life forces of a medicinal agent, and just as a glass has been known to crack when a certain chord is struck on a musical instrument, so the silver cord attaching the higher bodies to the coarser grained physical body in men, may snap across, if the most similar medicine is given in a very high potency.

THE LAWS GOVERNING THE SCIENCE AND THE BASIS OF THE REMEDIES

THE whole universe is governed by laws: Astronomy and Meteorology are based on the scientific calculations and laws of the mathematician and physicist; but Homo Sapiens himself is content to leave the treatment and cure of his bodily ailments to chance. Medicine and medical therapeutics are a law unto themselves by having no laws: Medicine is an art—you are told, and depends on the art of the diagnostician. Diagnosis is everything: find out what is wrong with the patient and the patient will be cured *ipso facto*! But is that really so? The same symptoms may be ascribed to antrum trouble, to a prolapsed kidney or kidneys, to a grumbling appendix, or to some phobia or repression of ideas in early childhood, according to whether you visit a rhinologist, a kidney enthusiast, a general surgeon or a psychologist. And after one or other of these organs have been excised, and the victim still feels ill, he may be sent from one surgeon to another and gradually be deprived of nearly all his organs and, still at the end of it all, he will not be one whit the better!

This has been so throughout the ages; only to mention the tale of the "woman with an issue of blood for twelve years and who had suffered many things of many physicians and had spent all that she had and was nothing bettered, but rather grew worse". (St. Mark V.)

We seem to have made very little progress since the days that Jesus walked in Galilee and performed his miracles.

Yes, the physician has concentrated on diagnosis and on the pseudo-scientific gadgets as an aid to diagnosis, and while the patient is being probed and tested, X-rayed and peered at through the bronchoscope and electric gastroscope and rectoscope and I don't know how many other scopes, what happens to the disease processes? What happens to the host, the owner of all these mysteries? methinks the patient himself is a secondary consideration.

Laboratory tests are regarded as of more importance than the individual, and observations at the bedside of the individual are rarely carried out nowadays. And yet laws exist to guide the physician how to treat the sick person; but unhappily they have never been officially recognized.

The first law is the law of simillimum, which is followed by (2) the principle of the minimum dose, (3) the principle of potentization. The statement "like cures like"—"Similia similibus curentur"—was first pronounced by Paracelsus, later re-discovered by Hahnemann, who then proceeded to build upon this fact his superstructure of scientific treatment by medicinal substances. Any substance, it may be of animal, vegetable or mineral origin, will produce certain reactions or symptoms, if given to the healthy individual for a long enough period. These reactions were collected by Hahnemann and his pupils, some 50 co-workers, mostly doctors, with great care and diligence—and the corollary followed : these self-same symptoms, if found in a sick person, would be removed or cured by the medicinal substance which produced them in the healthy individual. Let me give an example or two as proof of this contention :

The effects of a bee's sting—the virus of the honeybee, are well known : burning, stinging, lancinating pains with excessive swelling which come on rapidly and spread rapidly—hot applications make the burning, stinging pains worse—constitutional symptoms are occasionally produced in the involuntary prover or victims. There may be stiffness, constriction, difficulty in breathing, restlessness and general widespread œdema. If you find a sick person showing these symptoms, it may be in rheumatism, kidney disease, peritonitis, meningitis, you will be able to cure the disease with minute doses of *Apis* or bee virus.

There is a certain spider, called the black spider, which lurks in the underground passages and cellars of houses in Cuba and southern states of North America, and whose bite is much feared by the natives, not because it is painful. The person bitten does not realize that anything is wrong until the next day, when an inflamed pimple is seen, surrounded by a scarlet blush; this pimple continues to swell and spread, chill and fever sets in, the pimple becomes a large hard abscess which ends by mortification of the integuments over it and several small openings form which discharge a thick, sanious matter. In delicate children the bite may even prove fatal. The above condition resembles a carbuncle, and if you find carbuncles in patients, you may be quite certain that you will be able to disperse them rapidly with a few minute doses of the poison of the black spider or *Tarentula cubensis*, which has been used successfully in this manner in the past by physicians all over the world.

A third example: the bite of the Spanish spider—*Tarentula hispanica*—is followed by a dancing mania. After a bite dyspnœa, suffocation, blackness of the skin of the body comes on. If music is played, movement of the feet and hands and then the whole body is produced, violent dancing follows, and then the blackness of the face and hands goes off and the patient recovers. Curiously enough, every succeeding year at the same season the pain and attending symptoms recur, and they can always be averted by music. Therefore, if you get a patient with restlessness, chorea, hysteria, alternately laughing and crying, then think of *Tarentula hispanica*; it will cure certain types of hysteria or mental diseases in people who pretend or who feign chorea or twitching or go in for violent dancing when they know they are observed; but show no hysteria when unobserved or left alone. If these choreic or hysterical paroxysms are improved by music, then the Spanish spider in minute doses will effect a cure.

Atropa belladonna, the attractive black berries of the deadly nightshade, are often the cause of serious poisoning in children. These berries dilate the pupils of the eyes: the skin becomes dry and bright red, the face becomes scarlet, in fact, frequently cases of belladonna poisoning have been mistaken for cases of scarlatina, and therefore certain types of scarlet fever, the typical cases of Sydenham's scarlet, when the skin presents a smooth, even red surface, are cured by *Belladonna* within a day or two. "Give *Belladonna*", one doctor wrote some years ago, "and there was no need to notify scarlet or send them to the hospital. The next day, the rash and sore throat had disappeared." During an epidemic of scarlet fever it is a wise precaution to give *Belladonna* two or three times a day to all the children who are exposed to infection, and there will be no further spread.

The law of simillimum was tested out and proved by Hahnemann and his followers more than 130 years ago. Provings, as he called these experimental tests, were made, not on animals, as they are so frequently made in these days, but on healthy human beings. A number of individuals, men and women, were chosen, their peculiarities were noted, and for some days they received blank pills or powders; then a medicinal substance was added without their knowledge, and any reactions or symptoms that were produced were noted down, and a record was drawn up for each remedy proved. Cases of poisoning were collected from medical literature and their symptoms analysed and added to the record. If several provers produced the same symptom, that meant that this particular symptom would stand high and was certain to cure the same symptom in a sick person, and one of the first to be considered. In that way nearly 106 medicinal substances were proved at that time, and since Hahnemann's day a good many of these remedies have been re-proved, and the symptoms produced were found to be correct, and many other remedies have been more or less thoroughly tested and proved on healthy persons. So now we possess a Materia Medica of approximately 2,000 remedies from which to choose according to the law of similars the correct remedy for each case.

The law of the minimum dose followed on the law of the simillimum. Hahnemann found that if he gave the correctly indicated remedy in a case, say *Belladonna*, for a case of scarlet fever, he would produce violent reactions in the sick person. The patient was so sensitive to the correct remedy that physiological doses upset him, therefore he proceeded to try out smaller and smaller doses; and he tried them out with mathematical precision. He diluted each medicine first on the centesimal scale and later on, his pupil, Dr. Hering, introduced the decimal scale of potentization of drugs. Physicians on the Continent prefer the decimal scale of preparation as a rule; Hahnemann only employed the centesimal scale and found that a patient sensitized by the inherent disease products in his own body reacted favourably, that is, his symptoms were removed and he was consequently cured—by minutest or minimum doses of the curative remedy.

The method of preparing each medicine was roughly as follows; and right up to date we still carry on in the same fashion —as it cannot be improved upon :

A medicine is measured, one part of a drug is taken and is diluted with either 9 parts or 99 parts of the diluent vehicle, an inert or non-medicinal substance, usually sugar of milk or rectified spirit in the good old pre-war days. The drug is rubbed down for an hour in a porcelain mortar, if solid, with sugar of milk— triturated is the official term—by hand originally, nowadays by machine—until the medicinal substance is well incorporated into the diluent vehicle. This is your 1st centesimal. One part of this mixture is taken and again diluted and triturated for an hour with 9 or 99 parts of sugar of milk, according to whether you wish to use it on the decimal or centesimal scale : this makes the 2nd decimal or 2nd centesimal dilution or trituration : once again you take one part of this mixture and dilute with 9 or 99 parts of sugar of milk, triturate it carefully by hand for an hour, and this produces the 3rd decimal or 3rd centesimal dilution. After that all further dilutions as a rule are carried out with rectified spirit, or distilled water, or water and spirit. That is, one part of the mixture is diluted with 9 or 99 parts of alcohol or distilled water, or water and alcohol, and well shaken, and this makes the 4th decimal or the 4th centesimal potency, and so on. You can dilute as often as you like : Hahnemann found that by carrying out these procedures and on administering these drugs in this form that the action of the remedy was remarkably and definitely increased. He called it homœopathic action, as a drug can only act homœopathically if it is chosen according to the law of similars—according to the principle that like cures like.

A minute dose or infinitesimal dose does not make it a homœo-pathic dose or give it a homœopathic action : the remedy must be chosen also according to the selectivity of action—according to the principle that like cures like. These homœopathic solutions and attenuations were called potencies by Hahnemann as he found to his great surprise that they acted more powerfully than the ordinary solutions, not prepared with such mathematical precision and such minute care as regards exact dilution and definite trituration and succussion. This trituration or succussion is a most important part of the process of preparation of the drug, as without it the physical action of the breaking up of the molecules into ions could not take place.

Animal, vegetable or mineral substances when potentized are rendered more potent—not less, just because of this breaking up of their minutest particles, and this disintegration of their atoms by which their energy is liberated acts by releasing radio-active power.

You will say there can be nothing left after these substances have been so divided and subdivided except sugar of milk or water.

In the earlier days Hahnemann and his followers depended on

clinical tests and clinical cures, but we can show by scientific means that active remnants of medicinal substances are present in these triturations. For example, the spectroscope proves quite definitely the presence of active substances in the 9th centesimal dilutions, this was shown in 1862! In 1914 a French observer in Paris demonstrated the presence of copper in a 100th centesimal dilution.

Much research has since been done by Dr. W. E. Boyd in Glasgow. He worked with an insoluble metal and found that a spectrogram of the *Aurum metallicum* in the 7th decimal or $7x$ tincture showed definite presence of gold. He also proved that marked physical activity was present with $6x$ and $7x$ tinctures of *Radium bromide* and that electroscopic tests showed activity with the $10x$ preparations.

The power of the infinitesimal is being acknowledged by well-known exponents of the orthodox school : Langdon Brown spoke recently of the potency of the infinitesimal dose in the therapeutics of hormones and vitamins : for example, one part of the posterior lobe of the pituitary dissolved in 15,000 million parts of water can still produce contractions of the uterus, that is, one grain in 1,000 tons of fluid.

These are some short remarks on the principles of Homœopathy, but personal experience is necessary to convince one of the efficacy of its teaching.

THE ACTION OF THE MINIMUM DOSE IN ACUTE EPIDEMICS

SOME years ago there was a heated discussion in the Council Chambers of one of the northern cities on the pros and cons of Homœopathy and the advisability of giving the Homœopaths of the town access to beds and permission to practise in the local fever hospitals : one side stated in all sincerity that Homœopaths *might do no harm* in minor troubles, but that such severe maladies as measles and its complications, diphtheria and pneumonia required "skilled medical care and the administration of proper drugs and remedies". It would mean exposing the patients to greater danger, and the death rate would rise, if such heretics as Homœopaths were allowed to treat them. What the outcome was of this discussion, one does not know. Let us, however, examine these statements : What minor diseases are there which might be left safely to the care of Homœopaths? Is it not a well recognized fact that a neglected cold may quickly develop into a fatal broncho-pneumonia in thirty-six to forty-eight hours? that an apparently mild tonsillitis may suddenly become virulent and kill the patient in a few days; that a blister of the heel casually overlooked has been known to cause death in three or four days; and so on. Is a Homœopath even competent enough to recognize the seriousness of a condition so that he can call in a more learned brother when he feels a "minor" case is beyond him?

Are there no records of the results of Homœopathy in acute diseases? One trained nurse told me that in a fever hospital where she worked for some time, a homœopathic physician attended regularly, and though they used to laugh at his glasses of water and the tiny pilules he dissolved in it, the fact remained that his cases developed no complications; they went out in record time and deaths were almost unknown!—thus the testimony of an independent trained observer.

Let me quote chapter and verse for results in some epidemics in the past which were treated by Homœopaths and which can be verified, if so desired, in the archives of the particular towns and hospitals respectively. In 1813 there raged an epidemic of what was called war typhus in Central Europe, it might have been typhoid for all we know; these two diseases had not been pathologically and bacteriologically differentiated at that time, and thousands died under orthodox treatment or, in spite of treatment. In Leipzig there practised then one Samuel Hahnemann, the Father of this new school of treatment, based on the Law of Similars. He treated 183 cases of typhus, in accordance with his principles; he gave *Bryonia* in the 12th centesimal dilution to some cases, to others who presented slightly different symptoms he gave *Rhus tox.* 12th centesimal potency in infrequent drop doses. These were cases in the first stage of the disease. To those cases who progressed to the second stage, he prescribed *Hyoscyamus* in 8th or 9th dilution. And how many do you think survived the heroic measures of this heretic homœopath Hahnemann? 182 survived to tell the tale and only one died, and he was a very old, enfeebled person. You can read all about it in the newspapers of that period; for Hahnemann made no mystery of it, he explained everything clearly in his article; he went fully into the preparation of each remedy, and the reasons for giving the different medicines, so that other doctors could imitate him and repeat his success. So you see how successful Homœopathy proved itself in such a virulent and fatal disease as typhus, the mortality rate of which is well over 50 per cent. even now.

I can hear unbelievers say, of course, the diagnosis was wrong in the cases treated by Hahnemann, and these people who recovered did not have typhus at all: but the symptoms were carefully noted down in full and these records have been kept, and they are identical with the case histories of those of the orthodox physicians, and one can be absolutely certain that they were definitely serious cases of typhus.

And what is the record of the modern physician with all his latest equipments, bacteriological laboratories, serums and inoculations? Have we advanced at all in Medicine? at any rate as regards the recovery rate of serious epidemics?

I am not talking in a slighting spirit: I am only mentioning facts which stare one in the face. In 1937 we had an epidemic of typhoid here in England, 282 cases were notified and twenty-five deaths were reported as due to this disease so far, at the time of writing, and some more cases are said to be dangerously ill, and further cases may still end fatally. Therefore the death rate of typhoid these modern days is at least 8 per cent, or 80 per 1,000—and typhoid is not such a fatal or virulent disease as typhus! The homœopathic death rate in 1813 was .5 per cent. or 5 per 1,000 for the more fatal disease of typhus; the orthodox death rate is more than ten times as much! Figures speak!*

Unfortunately Homœopaths were not called in to treat the cases of typhoid. Oh, the pity thereof!

Now let us consider another epidemic disease; this time it shall be Asiatic cholera which raged in England in 1854. The results under allopathy showed a death rate of 59.2 per cent.; while the Homœopaths had a mortality rate of 16.4 per cent.; the percentage of recoveries among the Homœopaths was three times as great as the recovery rate in the orthodox hospitals. This unpleasant fact of the superiority of homœopathic over orthodox treatment was carefully suppressed, though a medical commission was sent to the London Homœopathic Hospital and their records were carefully scrutinized by a medical inspector, who certified them as correct. And these results are still being ignored. Nowhere in the medical textbooks do you see it mentioned that cholera treated homœopathically is not so fatal and has a higher recovery rate than orthodox allopathic treatment.

This conspiracy of silence still persists. The orthodox school will hardly investigate our claims that we can and do cure acute diseases more rapidly, without any subsequent complications than the recognized Medicine of the day. If a case recovers under homœopathic treatment, one usually hears it said that it was only a mild case, and it would have recovered anyhow!

And what about influenza? We have mild epidemics of it every year, and every thirty years or so a virulent type of influenza arrives and sweeps over the four quarters of the globe, ravaging and killing people by the thousand. The last epidemic, still within living memory, was of course in 1918, when many people among the war-wearied populations of the world were carried off. I do not know whether records are available of the mortality rate of influenza under homœopathic régime. I can only testify from personal experience to the invaluable help which homœopathic remedies gave me in treating the many cases of

* At the time of going to press, the figures according to the newspapers were as follows: 320 cases notified; with a total of 44 deaths. A mortality rate of 13.75%. And still it is not finished.

influenza under my care at that time. One treated over 100, nearer 150 cases; both rich and poor, young and old, male and female; and the results were astonishing. The cases were not picked ones; some were seriously ill when first seen, with high temperatures and bronchial involvement, some had it more mildly, and yet the temperatures in nearly all cases came down in twenty-four to forty-eight hours : they were kept strictly in bed for a week after the temperature was normal, kept on dilute fruit juices during the whole of the time—orange juice and grape juice, no milk, no tea was allowed. And there was not a single death in the whole of this series and no subsequent complications. The case that gave me most anxiety, and the only one which had a relapse within two weeks, and who remained ill altogether for six weeks, was a dispenser who insisted on trying out all the latest mixtures ordered by well-known physicians which were dispensed at her fashionable chemist's shop! The trouble I had with her, the temperature went up and up, various complications developed and I was afraid she was going to slip through my hands; how grateful I was when I could sign her off and get her away for a change of air at the seaside! After that I refused to allow any patient to order their own treatment, they had to obey my instructions or go somewhere else.

One's cases were not particularly mild at the start, and yet they one and all said when they recovered, "What a mild attack I had." They did not grasp that the innocuous looking medicine had anything to do with their rapid recovery. *Arsenic* in minutest doses was the remedy that proved most helpful in many of these cases; but that does not mean that *Arsenic* would always answer in every epidemic of influenza. You have to find the picture of the epidemic, which varies from season to season. In moist warm seasons most cases would be covered by *Gelsemium*; in dry cold, windy weather, *Aconite and Nux vomica* would come in, and so forth. The curious part of the 1918 influenza epidemic was this : twenty years later I read in an American journal that *Arsenic was the epidemic* remedy in *America* in 1918. Homœopathic physicians cannot help agreeing with one another; the same *variety* of symptoms *mean the* same *drug* to them—that is what is meant by the Law of Similars. Do you get this among the Regulars? Almost every physician has his pet remedies, his pet mixtures, and if you would send round, as was done once by a wealthy man many years ago, a set of symptoms with a demand for a prescription to twenty different physicians, you would get twenty different prescriptions sent to you, unless you include any homœopathic doctors, and then you would—and *do*—get the same remedy for the same set of symptoms. This is true Science.

The therapeutic knowledge of doctors of medicine is unfortunately contracting more and more; they despise the many drugs handed down to them by their forefathers and only use the latest products of the vast drug combines, such as the sulphonamides for bacterial diseases or the latest drug, Penicillin, if the case should prove sulphonamide-resistant.

Sedatives of the aspirin or barbiturate group are freely prescribed on the flimsiest pretexts for all sorts of diseases. Thus there is certainly more therapeutic agreement among the doctors of the day than there was some decades ago. But is it not a fact also that new and terrible diseases follow after these modern cure-alls? The list of diseases caused by one of the 70 odd varieties of Sulphonamides is truly astounding.

The cure of acute diseases seems worse than the actual original disease itself. On the other hand, what do you find under homœopathic treatment?

Take whatever disease you like, whether infectious or otherwise; homœopathic physicians can—and do—deal with it promptly and judiciously, and as Hahnemann puts it in his *Organon*—his textbook of homœopathic philosophy—"This is the right and proper way to cure : the highest ideal of a cure is a rapid, gentle and permanent restoration of health or removal and annihilation of disease in its whole extent, with shortest, most reliable and most harmless way on comprehensible principles."

Not so very long ago a doctor in general practice, a recent convert to Homœopathy, was faced with a serious epidemic of measles in the little town he practised in. He applied the newly learned principles to his patients, and jubilantly wrote a little while afterwards of the unexpected and marvellous results he had : 300 measles cases cured in record time with no deaths and no complications ! Can orthodox medicine beat this?

Another doctor wrote that by giving *Belladonna* to his scarlet fever patients, the rash, sore throat and temperature disappeared within twenty-four hours, so that there was no need to notify these cases.

Again in diphtheria, Homœopaths have sent the throat swabs to the bacteriological laboratories for examination, and by the time the positive result came back, the throat had cleared up, the membrane had gone and the case was cured. There is a story of a nurse with a diphtheric throat being sent to the Fever Hospital when her swab was positive, after a dose of the indicated homœopathic remedy had been given. The next morning the Medical Officer rang up the Homœopathic Hospital to enquire whether a mistake had not been made, there was no sign of any diphtheria. He was then shown the positive bacteriological slide and had to believe the diagnosis which had been made on the strength of it and *nolens volens*! believe in the cure of the disease by Homœopathy.

Whooping cough also can be cut short by homœopathic remedies. I have seen it many times, and there are no complications, and the children after two to three weeks of whooping cough under this treatment look well and bonny! The homœo- pathic nosode or vaccine *Pertussin* or *Coqueluchinum*, which is the French name for this nosode, works exceedingly well in the minute doses. I have given it in suspected and actually defined cases; I have tried it in institutions to prevent a further spread and succeeded several times in limiting threatening outbreaks to the first one or two cases. Those irritating and lingering cases where the whoop persists long after the customary six weeks, and which as the old wives have it, will not stop "until May is out", clear up rapidly after a few doses of *Pertussin* in the 12th or 13th potency. So it works in all stages of the disease: it pre- vents, it shortens, and also stops late sequelae. It goes well with other whooping cough remedies, which may be needed as specific indications arise; and if you begin the control of this disease with this nosode, broncho-pneumonia does not arise, which is an ex- tremely fatal complication under orthodox treatment. The intense tickling of fauces and trachea which precedes the cough is soon lessened, the vomiting and nausea at the end of the cough is, as a rule, controlled within a week or two, and as a result meta- bolism is not interfered with and loss of weight and wasting does not take place—which would rob whooping cough of nearly all its terrors. In some early cases I have given one dose of *Drosera* 30th or 200th potency, and the disease stopped with miraculous suddenness; the chief characteristics of *Drosera* are: spasmodic cough, frequent spells of barking cough, worse evenings and after midnight, vomits if he cannot bring up even a little phlegm and violent tickling cough in larynx. It does not work in all cases of whooping cough; some cases have slightly different symptoms, and then other remedies are required : but *Pertussin* itself is as near a specific as can be found anywhere.

Mumps is another epidemic disease, which can be very unpleasant. No medicine is required according to the textbooks, even though there may be serious complications, and fatal cases have occurred. The best treatment I know for it homœopathically is a remedy highly praised by Dr. Burnett, this is *Pilocarpine*, which, given in the 6th dilution two or three times daily reduces the temperature in twenty-four to thirty-six hours, and diminishes the swelling of the parotid gland in forty-eight to seventy-two hours, so that before the week is out, the parotid gland is normal again. *Pilocarpine* is almost a specific for mumps and acts as an *"organ"* remedy on the parotid and sweat glands. We have been through an extensive, though mild, epidemic since July 1937, and all the thirty odd cases seen responded in the manner described; there were no complications in the series.

Last, but not least, there is pneumonia, one of the diseases specifically mentioned by the objectors to homœopathic treatment as being beyond the ken of the heretics. Professor Osler, in his *Principles and Practice of Medicine,* says that pneumonia is the most fatal of all acute diseases; killing more than diphtheria and outranking even consumption as a cause of death. Mortality ranges from 20 to 40 per cent. in orthodox hospitals, and it is specifically said that pneumonia is a *self-limited* disease *which can neither* be *aborted* nor cut *short by any known means at our command,* and again, there is no *specific treatment for pneumonia.* We were taught in Edinburgh that the physician was of very little use at the bedside of a pneumonia patient; that it *all depended on the nurse. Good nursing pulled a patient through; not the doctor's medicines.* What a to-do there was with a pneumonia case in the wards. Special nurses were put on and relieved every two to three hours, and each nurse looked after the one case only; half-hourly feeds were given and religiously charted; the patient's strength had to be kept up and supported; and what a triumph it was for the nurse, when on the ninth day the crisis occurred, and the patient's temperature dropped. Everything and everybody was hushed in the ward during these crucial moments. When I was house physician in a homœopathic hospital I told the visiting physician with bated breath that a case of right-sided pneumonia had been admitted to the ward, and was more than shocked that he treated it as quite an ordinary occurrence and I did not believe him, when he cheerfully said, "We shall cure her in less than a week"; and he spoke the truth. In five days the crisis occurred, and the patient went out very shortly afterwards! I do not pretend to be an authority on pneumonia; but the six cases of pneumonia I looked after in my practice all survived, so the percentage saved under homœopathic treatment was 100 per cent., or perhaps I was particularly lucky, and my six cases all belonged to the category of 80 out of every 100 that survive treatment. But they did not have any special nursing; these people were too poor; one could only send in a district nurse night and morning, so they were not saved by good nursing; survival was due to the action of the homœopathic medicaments they received.

Before me lies a book by two homœopathic physicians, Drs. A. and T. Pulford of Toledo in Ohio, America, called *Homœopathic Leaders in Pneumonia*. They state in their preface that they have been treating 242 *cases of pneumonia* of all *types and degrees of severity: some coming directly* from and *others having been confirmed* in the *diagnosis by allopaths with but three deaths: a rate of* 1.4 *per cent*. They say, that they can hardly understand a fixed minimum death rate of 25 per cent. much less a maximum death rate of 95 per cent. in a disease as readily amenable to the proper remedy as is pneumonia.

You can believe it or not! but seeing is believing—one has seen pneumonia cases having the crisis as early as the third day, and none were later than the fifth day.

So Osler is proved wrong : pneumonia *is and can be limited* and *can be cut short by the correctly indicated remedy*. Orthodox medicine has at last scored a bull in pneumonia and can triumphantly point to the reduction in the death rate of pneumonia since the use of various Sulphonamide preparations from the old rate of 20-40 deaths for 100 people attacked to the latest figures of 8 per cent. A great achievement, I admit, but their results are still not as good as the highest results amongst the cases of pneumonia treated at the Homœopathic Hospitals. In a series of 24,000 cases treated at these hospitals, the highest death rate was just about 5 per cent., and these included cases treated with serums; the purely homœopathically treated cases showed a death rate of 3 per cent. and one homœopathic doctor achieved a death rate of 1.5 per cent. in a series of several hundred cases.

Can somebody enlighten me why cases of pneumonia treated and cured with Sulphonamide so frequently develop a second and even a third attack within a few months? And why does it leave most of the individuals "cured" by it so weak that they require weeks of convalescence to get over the effects of the cure? And why do a large percentage develop other serious and hitherto unknown blood diseases after it? And why is it that a certain percentage die suddenly and unexpectedly, shortly after the supposed cure—of heart failure? Homœopathically treated cases do not show any of these complications.

Another example of the old saying, I suppose. "The disease was successfully treated, but the patient died."

HOMŒOPATHY IN DENTISTRY

AT the Dispensary some time ago a little girl was brought to my notice with a swollen face following a dental operation with the following symptoms: pain in jaw with stiffness and difficulty in opening the mouth. *Arnica* 30 in three or four doses was given to her, and she was asked to show herself to the dentist next morning. As I had predicted, the swelling had gone entirely, the socket of the extracted tooth was clean and not inflamed, as it had been the previous day, and the dental surgeon was much impressed with the rapidity of the cure. A week or two later the self-same dentist sent an S O S message to me: "Can you give me the medicine which cured the little girl so quickly? A private patient of mine has also got a swollen face, a great deal of pain and inability to open her mouth." A stock prescription of *Arnica* 6 was sent to her with instructions "to be used as often as the urgency of the individual case required and medicine to be stopped when the patient was feeling better". The dentist reported a few days later that the patient was extremely astonished and gratified with the almost instantaneous relief she experienced after taking one of these tasteless pills. "I could open my mouth within twenty minutes of taking the first dose, and I felt better after each dose I took. Much better than all the mouth washes, and I do not feel so ill either, as I usually do after the usual dopes."

Still a third example: this time to show that *Arnica* is just as efficacious in preventing bruising, as in removing it. A doctor's wife had several enormous fangs removed under a general anaesthetic. They proved to be rather more stubborn than was at first expected, and previous experience had taught my dentist friend that pain and an ugly disfigurement were bound to develop; so very diffidently, seeing this was a doctor's wife, she asked her whether her husband would mind her taking something which would prevent all this unnecessary suffering. Being reassured on this matter, she gave her *Arnica* 6, one pill, and asked her to come back in a couple of hours. Everything appeared normal, no swelling had occurred, so to make doubly sure, she offered her another pill of *Arnica*. "What is that, what are you giving her?" interjected her doctor husband. On being shown the bottle of *Arnica*, which was labelled, my lord exclaimed, "Oh! you can give her as much of *that* as you like, that won't make any difference." The dentist quietly remarked, "One pill will do, you will see." And he did see, the next morning his wife woke up having had no pain and minus any swelling. Did it convince the doctor? Oh, dear no, that was "just an accident, don't you know."

Hæmorrhages will occur, even in the best regulated dental surgeries, after extractions, and they are a great trial to everybody concerned, including anxious parents and frightened children. And the doctor who is called in, usually in the early hours of the morning, is naturally blaming the unfortunate dentist, and as for hospital house-surgeons, their language is more than lurid and illuminating, as to what they think of *that* dentist. Well, Homœopathy does not leave one high and dry, even during such emergencies as a dental cavity that simply won't stop bleeding. No need for packs or stitching up the cavity, or applying adrenalin, or any other violent method, as recommended by the highest authorities. All that is needed is a pill or two of *Phosphorus*, almost any potency, 6x, or 6, or 30 or even higher. The bleeding just stops, as if by a miracle after Phos.

I remember years ago being called to a case of dental hæmorrhage. Everywhere was gore, huge clots inside the mouth, the mother was weeping, as she thought her darling's last hour had come, and not absolutely sure whether a mere woman could be trusted to cope with a serious case, especially when all I did was to produce a case of medicine and pop a wee powder into the child's mouth. This was repeated every ten minutes, then every quarter of an hour and in an hour's time the mouth was nice and clean. The mother was quite impressed. As for the nurses, you should hear them on the subject of these pills. "Do they work? Of course they do, we should not like to be without them, they halve our anxiety and there are no anxious mothers sending up messages—'Is my child all right?'"

So I should advise all and sundry who fall into the dentist's hands to equip themselves with *Arnica* for pain and swelling, and with *Phosphorus* for any bleeding which may distress them subsequently, and the visit to the dentist will be robbed of half its fear and anxiety.

One remembers a rather alarming experience: a lady was obliged to have one of her lower teeth out and was given *Phosphorus* previously to prevent any bleeding, and I fancy, was told to take *Arnica* 30 in repeated doses afterwards to prevent pain and swelling. I was rung up in the afternoon and informed that she was bleeding profusely and had been told by the local doctor to go to hospital for its arrest and that probably suturing would be necessary. She wished for homœopathic treatment, so I went along prepared with my box of tricks, i.e. medicine case and surgical aids such as I thought I might require, needles, sutures, etc. On arrival I found a typical picture of a patient after severe hæmorrhage, pale exsanguinated, restless. On examination, I found oozing from the dental cavity and a spurting artery from underneath the tongue, evidently due to a laceration from the dental gag. It would have been a very difficult job to put a suture on the tongue without an anæsthetic, all on my own, as I was, and I felt tempted to give in and send it to the surgeon. Pressure applied for hours had not been sufficient to stop the bleeding. I tried *Phosphorus* 1m, a dose every ten minutes, it stopped the bleeding from the cavity of the tooth, but not the bleeding from the lacerated tongue. Was Homœopathy no good after all? I remembered this patient was ordinarily a *Lachesis* patient, this was her constitutional remedy, and this snake virus from the Surukuku snake of South America had been proved to act well in hæmorrhages: so *Lachesis* 30 was given. Almost immediately after the first dose the bleeding slackened, became paler and coagulation took place in the spurting artery. I saw it myself before my very eyes! Of course it was only a very small artery, it is true—I repeated the *Lachesis* in fifteen minutes, but coagulation was complete in ten minutes. I waited for some time, in case there should be a recurrence: the cure held good, and except for exhaustion and weariness and a swollen lower jaw, it was inevitable that there should be swelling, after all the manipulations the poor lady had put up with: the patient had no bad after-effects. Rest in bed and further doses of *Lachesis* finished this adventure. One was grateful again for the power that Homœopathy gave in such an alarming case as hæmorrhage always is. There are many hæmorrhage remedies, and the wise physician will carefully memorize all the symptoms of each one: this knowledge will stand him in good stead in an emergency.

Coffea is another remedy which may be required after dental extraction. These are highly excitable, nervous people, who find pain unbearable; there is the constant cry "Do not touch me. I cannot bear you to come near me." They feel the very vibrations of the floor boards from anyone walking across it. Wide awake all night, extremely restless, increased sensibility to touch, jar, noise and light. Feel the cold very much, worse cold wind, sensitive to fresh air and to draughts. Yet with all this pain in the jaws and the mouth, there is relief from holding cold water in the mouth; the colder the better. Cannot drink warm tea or touch warm food, without its making the pains much worse.

It is astounding how quickly the pain and swelling disappear in those hypersensitive people after a few doses of *Coffea*, even in such low potencies as 3x or 6x.

HOMŒOPATHY IN OBSTETRICS

MANY people have the mistaken idea that a pregnant woman is a sick woman, and should be treated as such, and take great care of herself—while the very opposite is, or should be, the case.

Nature has so arranged matters that metabolism is increased during that time, more blood is carried to the reproductive organs, and the circulation is improved, and a child-bearing woman should look, and be, at her best. The curious part is : that hidden constitutional errors show themselves during that period, and therefore the best time to give real, worth-while constitutional treatment is during the nine months in which a mother is bearing her child. There would be great benefit, not only to the mother, but also to the child; two individuals are raised to a higher state of normal good health, and thus not only the individual, but eventually the whole race, could be improved.

What a tremendous field of activity lies before the Homœopaths, if they are given the chance! Antenatal clinics are helpful, so far as they go, but they only diagnose and point out anything that is wrong; the actual treatment is negligible.

Diet, of course, is of the greatest importance during this time; the old wives' saying is : "a mother should feed for two"—but this is entirely fallacious. One girl followed this advice with her first baby, and stuffed herself : lived on the fat of the land; rested frequently on the sofa, and did not take any exercise, or do any work in the house. The result was an immense boy of 15 lbs., an extremely slow, difficult labour; instruments; the mother was badly torn—and the baby died two days later of cerebral hæmorrhage.

An infant's weight can be regulated by the mother's diet. The best weight to arrive at for an easy labour is round about 6 lbs. These are lean babies, it is true, but there will not be a preliminary loss of weight, as there is commonly, in heavier babies, during the first week; the infant starts to put on weight from the first.

The best diet during pregnancy is a strict lacto-vegetarian-fruitarian diet from at least three months onwards. If the mother cannot do without the fleshpots, fish two or three times a week up to six months might be allowed; on the whole it is better to forgo all fish, flesh, or fowl, of any kind.

The reward is great; the mother feels well; there will be no trouble during the actual labour; no instruments will be necessary; labour will be easy and short; the baby will be small, lean and compact; the head is soft and easily compressible, and it is a healthy baby, invariably. This has been proved to the writer's satisfaction throughout a period of twenty years; seventeen years in general practice, and many years as Medical Officer of an Ante-natal Clinic—*provided* the mother carries out the instructions given her.

It is difficult, of course, to convince the ordinary working-class mother that meat is unnecessary, and that she will not feel weak if she discontinues it; hence, the best results were obtained with sensible, middle-class parents, who understood one's reasons, and faithfully followed instructions.

To particularize, briefly, diet should be on these lines : wholemeal bread, porridge, whole bran, eggs in moderation—not more than one a day—and at least one pint of milk, daily. Any kind of vegetables, conservatively cooked or steamed; raw salads—at least one, daily. Even in England, salads are obtainable all the year round, and at a reasonable cost, if you are content with watercress, celery or tomatoes, swedes, parsnips, shredded and grated carrots, turnips, hearts of cabbage, sprouts and cauliflower, during the winter. Fruit there is, in variety; apples, oranges, grapefruit, lemons, prunes, dates, figs; all soft fruits, in season, as much as can be taken; nuts, if well masticated, or grated in a nut-mill. For cereals, tapioca, rice, etc., and use Barbados sugar, not bleached white sugar. Finally include wholemeal macaroni, cheese—preferably freshly-made cream cheeses— and you have a varied and interesting diet which is easily digestible. No meat juices, of course, should be used; only Marmite and similar vegetable extracts, for flavouring purposes.

This diet has been tried out effectively even in the cases of women round about the age of forty, and the confinements were easy, and caused no anxiety.

No coffee and no stimulants should be taken, tea only in strict moderation, and no other liquids except water, milk, barley water and fruit juices.

Homœopathy should be the only medicinal treatment. As I

have said before—the health of an expectant mother can be wonderfully benefited during this time, and if a woman feels well during pregnancy, though ailing between her confinements, the precept of simple remedies and simple living will have been driven home, and have its favourable repercussions in raising the standard of general health in the community.

A prescription of *Psorinum* during pregnancy will improve her general health after the birth of the child.

The writer recalls, some time ago, being asked to watch over a confinement case from the beginning. This was a lady who had previously been her patient, and been treated for anæmia and pretubercular debility. She looked unhealthy, pale and pasty, with greasy skin and hair, and a spotty face; buxom and well-developed, with too much fat on her body. Town life never suited her, she declared; she always felt tired and done-up : very sleepy; in character she was reserved, somewhat sullen and sulky. A few doses of *Calc. carb.* 30, and later *Tuberculinum*, helped to bring colour to her cheeks.

Then she decided to marry, and have a child, if she could be treated homœopathically all the time. I made a pact with the husband that no allopathic drugs, and no antiseptics were to be used. I was willing to try the experiment, even though we had been trained to use all sorts of strong lotions, etc., in midwifery practice.

The patient was put on a very strict diet from about two months onwards, and persisted with it bravely; her health improved greatly. Round about five months she developed some symptoms of indigestion, and mental symptoms—aversion to her husband, irritability, fits of temper; threatened to do herself an injury during one of these turns; was indifferent whether she had a baby or not, and so forth. She was given *Sepia xm.*, and the irritability, temper and indifference disappeared. Life was sweet and pleasant once more, she found! A little later there was some colic and abdominal pain, and slight constipation, with the sensation of drawing like a string from the navel—which *Plumbum* 30 removed. Nothing further of interest developed, except that she lost weight, her looks improved, and she felt well. Then the great day arrived. I had sufficient faith in Homœopathy to feel that everything would go well, even though the orthodox mid-wives were shocked at the absence of all antiseptics; no lysol, no dettol at all; no mercurial lotions! They cast their eyes Heavenwards; and thought we were slightly demented—and feared that everything would go wrong. We, of course, took all aseptic precautions; had plenty of boiling water and aseptic dressings, with gloves, coats and surgically clean towels, etc.

The actual labour lasted less than eighteen hours, from beginning to end; very good—for a first baby! During the second stage she developed some symptoms of restlessness; the pains were slow and ineffective; she threw herself about, would not lie on her back; flung off her clothes, complaining of heat; wanted the windows open; could not endure any more! One dose of *Pulsatilla high,* and she settled down serenely, and the pains became more powerful.

The baby, a nice boy, arrived without any trouble, and as there was some hæmorrhage, *Arnica* was given, which quickly settled the bleeding and brought down the placenta. There was a slight tear, unfortunately, owing to the broad shoulders of the boy, and we had to put in two or three stitches. *Arnica* internally, and *Calendula* lotion, externally, sprayed neat on to the perineum, and dressings moistened in diluted *Calendula* lotion, applied outside, hastened the healing process. We had no rise in temperature, no malaise; bowels moved easily; after three days the breast milk came in quite normally, and we had no anxiety the whole time. Nor was there any sign of sepsis; everything healed beautifully and soundly, without fuss or unnecessary interference, left to the good offices of Nature. Incidentally, the midwife was astonished to find how quickly the perineum healed with *Calendula,* and how little vaginal discharge there was.

In another case, where everything appeared to be going satisfactorily up to a few days before labour set in, the husband wished to have the best "specialist" possible; forthwith the patient was sent into the private wards of a teaching hospital.

There she suffered a fractured rib; labour was slow and delayed, and she was given various injections to hasten matters; then there was extensive laceration, a rise in temperature, threatened pyæmia. Subsequently, there was backache, lasting for months, and a chronic vaginal discharge remained behind for nearly a year—until the patient recommenced homœopathic treatment. This removed the backache and leucorrhœa, which was due to congestion of the uterus, but not until she had taken *Fraxinus americana* and a few doses of *Sepia,* did the trouble finally clear up. No douches should be used in such cases; the less interference there is, the better for the patient.

In the writer's view, the increasing hospitalization of maternity cases is wrong. The patients are taken from their accustomed surroundings into the wards, where there is likely to be a concentration of septic germs, and the danger of septic infection is much greater. In America, where nearly every mother goes into hospital to have her baby, the maternal death rate is nearly double—and some years more than double—that in England.

In consequence, in the past year or two, there has been something of a *volte face*, and mothers are being advised to arrange for their confinements in their own homes.

Let me instance, however, a maternity home in South London where in 15,000 births there has not been a single maternal death!

From the beginning the mothers are carefully instructed in the principles and practice of vegetarian dietary, and required to follow it during the period of pregnancy and lying-in.

Again, in one of the southern suburbs of London, there is a maternity home combining Homœopathy with fruitarian and vegetarian diet, and here also there have been no maternal deaths.

Notwithstanding, many obstetric specialists declare that diet in the pre-natal period makes no difference at all; that a mixed diet is necessary for the well-being of mother and child.

Time proves all things, and slowly but surely, the meatless diet in pregnancy should come into its own! Variety enough is offered in the garnered wealth of Mother Earth herself—sun-ripened fruit and grain, nutritious roots, coming to slow maturity above and below the soil in the ordered sequence of their seasons.

And how much illness, how much anxiety and discomfort could be averted if womankind, generally adopted a rational health diet, coupled with homœopathic treatment, in pregnancy. The birth rate would rise and the nation be potentially wealthier in a rising generation of sturdy children. There would be less neurosis, fewer nervous and physical wrecks, with childbirth bereft of its terrors; with healthy, happy periods of pregnancy. Our mothers would not dread their confinements, and the all-round gain to the community would be incalculable.

The maternal death rate in Great Britain has dropped from 4.2 per 1,000 at which figure it had stayed for years, to 2.5 per

1,000 in the last four years, nearly half of the rate of what it was before 1939. And the great alteration has been the change in the diet. The pregnant mothers get a priority ration of 1 pint of milk per day; they get extra orange juice and an issue of cod-liver oil and three eggs per week, and owing to the shortage of meat and fish, they have to live chiefly on a diet of vegetables.

And again, it is of interest to note that the birth rate has risen steeply; many more people consume raw vegetable stuff, both raw green leaves and raw grated roots. The dietetic chemists have discovered that green leaves contain a large proportion of vitamin E, which increases the fertility rate. Have not the theories I propounded above proved to be true in praxis?

But, I suppose, as soon as meat, fish, etc., will become plentiful, the lessons learnt in this war will be forgotten and everybody will return to the fleshpots.

And against this "Back to Nature" method as advocated by Homœopathy, consider the thousands of pounds spent on research laboratories, in the endeavour to find the cause of maternal sepsis—the dread germ would promptly become innocuous, if the mothers could be induced by right food and simple living, these natural correctives, to forge their own armour against the onset of disease. Forget about the bacteria, they are only the scavengers of the disease, not the cause of the disease, help to eliminate them by a clean diet of fruit juices and the correct homœopathic remedy, and do not use any chemicals and drugs made from coal tar and aniline dyes which are uncertain, and sometimes deadly, in their action.

There is a book on *Homœopathy in Obstetrics* by Dr. Guernsey, which may appropriately be mentioned here. On some counts it may be regarded as "old-fashioned," but I should not like to be without it. It is most helpful, and covers all the eventualities, showing also, that much operative interference might be saved if the right homœopathic remedies were applied, and thus much morbidity, and possible fatalities, could be avoided.

Scattered over Great Britain and Ireland, the Continent, and the United States, there are medical men and women who have proved by clinical experience the advantages of Homœopathy in maternity work and the production of healthy offspring; and in succeeding generations, one hopes that ultimately the homœopathic principles may be universally applied.

HOMŒOPATHY IS THE BEST PREVENTIVE

PREVENTION is in the air; nutrition clinics are springing up; milk and extra nourishment are provided free or for next to nothing to expectant mothers; free advice on all kinds of health topics is broadcast on the wireless: but as always, the surest and safest kind of prevention is being ignored: Homœopathy. It may be a controversial topic, but I know this: that along with simple and conservatively cooked vegetables; some raw food daily, such as salads which are always available in some form or other all the year round; and fruit, wholemeal bread and only a modicum of meat and fish—homœopathic treatment would prevent many illnesses which come on in old age or even at an earlier stage—that is in the forties and fifties. In looking back over the decades one can recall several instances of people one has kept in contact with for anything from eighteen to twenty years, where one has watched their medical histories:

There is No. 1, who is a member of a decent-sized family, four girls and two boys; she is the eldest and has had homœopathic treatment for nigh on eighteen years, with only a very short break in between. She has been subject to lumbago and sciatica, which when treated allopathically, crippled her for well over a fortnight; the next dose of rheumatism she had she was treated "scientifically" according to the homœopathic principles with *Rhus. Tox.* and *Bryonia*, and it only incommoded her for two or three days. A non-meat diet for a month prevented a recurrence.

Severe colds and influenzal bronchitis were another trouble, always coming on early in January, and keeping her at home for a couple of weeks or so, and leaving her with a cough of several weeks' duration with pain and aching at the right base of the lungs, until she was asked to report at the first warning of the enemy, when *Carbo vegetabilis* or *Bryonia* or *Ipecacuanha* in repeated doses would soon clear up the influenza and even prevent the spread to the lungs. *Kali carb.*, as a constitutional remedy, when seen the first time at the end of the influenzal attack—cleared up the right-sided, undissolved pneumonia in a remarkably quick time.

But the greatest bugbear in the daily life of this lady was the menstrual suffering, the drenching periods, the pain and the excessive tiredness and exhaustion during this time. She received various remedies, *Ipecac.* and *Sepia* most frequently, whenever necessary. For a whole year she was seen weekly after an accident to her right ankle, a very severe sprain of the ankle ligaments and ankle joint, which threw the locomotor organs out of gear for many weeks : foot and leg muscles and the hips were crippled, and for months she limped. However, *Arnica*, followed by *Rhus. tox.*, *Ruta* and later *Calc. carb.*, all in repeated doses along with regular massage, manipulations and radiant light and re-education of the muscles by means of the Bristow electric coil, made a sound job of the torn ligaments and stretched muscles; and there is now a perfect joint, no limp; no recurrent rheumatism reminds her of the old accident. Homœopathy and physical therapy removed all that. Now she has gone through the menopause easily and comfortably, without any distress—in fact, she had no trouble at all. She feels better than she has done for years, and well able for a hard day's work. She has hardly any grey hairs, and looks years younger than her age. Her mother confesses she is surprised how well she looks, and that she herself at that age was always ailing and always seedy.

Now the interesting part is to compare this lady's health with that of her three sisters. They all had trouble with their periods; heavy losses, pain, etc. The one sister developed an ovarian cyst and had all the generative organs removed; the other sister had fibroids and had a large portion of the uterus— and the rest—cut out. The youngest now is going the same way, she has been or is being curetted previous to a doubtful tumour? Is it coincidence that the only one who had homœopathic treatment escaped the operations her sisters had? She herself knows and gives praise where it is due : to Homœopathy, and is thankful that she escaped all the trouble and pain, and worse, following an operation.

If this were the only case, one *might* say, it was a coincidence : but one hears it again and again, and one reads how homœopathic physicians save their patients from the operating table; and while doing so, prevent chronic invalidism and turn the patients into much stronger and healthier individuals: true prevention indeed!

The lady I have just been talking about, has for years now followed the diet described previously, eats freely of green vegetables, drinks the vegetable water, partakes of salads and fruit daily, and enjoys therefore excellent health, and is an advertisement to Homœopathy *and proper diet.*

No. 2 was a younger woman, when she became a convert, at first unknowingly, until she experienced the benefits of Homœopathy and became a devotee. She was thin and delicate and always suffering from colds and chills, which swiftly developed into influenza. In fact, she was one of the kind who always had a clinical thermometer close at hand; it was as much a necessity to her as the powder puff for her shiny nose. Early on, she insisted on being given a course of anti-catarrhal vaccines which apparently for a season or two prevented these severe chills; but when she was taken firmly in hand and had regular treatment with the sugar pills, there was very little doubt in her mind that Homœopathy acted with greater certainty than the old way of treatment. In fact, she expected to get well in twenty-four or at least forty-eight hours, and usually it was so. The only time she was ill for three weeks was when, during the holidays, she developed an attack of mumps with a temperature of 104 degrees for days, and was kept severely in bed and sweated and purged by a "regular." Much to her disgust her family would not hear of anything except the local doctor's treatment, as they preferred his nostrums to Homœopathy. The result was she came back to town thoroughly weakened and suffered from extreme depression and mucous colitis for months: this depression is a common sequel of mumps, whether due to the treatment or to the mumps itself, I do not know. All I know is, that homœopathic treatment of mumps does not produce this depression. One has just had experience of a minor epidemic of mumps, and not one of the children developed it, and they were well in less than a week. But this is by the by, and the full story will be told another time, I hope.

Lady No. 2 left with colitis and depression after the mumps incident, had specimens taken of the excreta and Bacillus Morgan being found, a homœopathic preparation was made of it in the 30th and 200th dilutions, and after a course of this remedy followed by *Pulsatilla* 30 and 200, she recovered completely after three months from both colitis and depression. Her recovery was not exactly helped favourably by hair-raising tales of all her acquaintances of the various cases of colitis they knew of, who had been ill for years, some five, some ten, some eighteen years, without any prospect of relief. Yet Homœopathy conquered again, and in three months she was well of her colitis. Another of this lady's trials was the monthly period; the dysmenorrhœa and the nausea and vomiting and collapse were always very exhausting every month. Various remedies were required, *Colocynth, Nux vomica* and *Ipecac.* were of the greatest help at various times; in fact, *Ipecacuanha* was a constant stand-by, until constitutional treatment with *Pulsatilla, Calcarea* and *Lycopodium* produced painless and easy periods—a great relief to a woman who has got to earn her living. She has developed physically and mentally in the last fifteen years, since she got to know of this disease-preventing treatment, and has gained well over two stones in weight and is at the top of her form; not always tired and sick and exhausted, continually complaining and ailing.

No. 3 has only had an eleven years' record with homœopathic treatment, the first contact was during an attack of German measles, which only lasted a very few days, and she was back at her job in ten days, after repeated doses of *Pulsatilla* and *Sulphur.* An excellent record; one knows that during the Great War, hundreds of women in Government offices developed German measles, and they were ill, sometimes for weeks; and some even died. German measles is not a joke in a grown-up person and can make one seriously ill. Afterwards it was discovered that this lady was a very rheumatic subject, always liable to rheumatism in her limbs and rheumatic throats, which came on during and after wet weather; *Rhus. tox.* 6 was prescribed because of this rheumatic basis, and it wrought better than she thought possible. These throats used to make each winter a very unpleasant time, a season to be dreaded; one winter even, she was in bed for quite a long period and away from her work for many days.

After taking *Rhus tox.* the throats used to disappear quickly; so that she got into the habit of keeping a stock of *Rhus tox.* at her home and taking a dose or two at the first premonitory sign with very happy results. She remarked the other day that she had not spent a day in bed for over eleven years and had never been off duty all that time! She had a touch of a septic throat some summers ago which was different from the usual rheumatic affliction. It was a septic condition; the tonsils were inflamed, dark red in colour and huge, entirely painless, even though they were so inflamed. *Baptisia* seemed to improve at first, but it was only after one discovered the great tenderness on the outside, the fear of being touched, the aggravation from a jar and from turning the head, that one recognized *Belladonna*, and *Bell.* two or three doses rapidly cleared up this throat. Her constitutional drug was *Silica*, and she responded very nicely to it. Even as a child and right up to date, she had a tendency to slip and fall to the ground; her body bore many marks of these humiliating experiences, especially her poor knees were always in the wars. She felt the cold very much and loathed the winters, as they made her feel so miserable, and psychologically, she was diffident, somewhat lacking in confidence, kept herself in the background, was afraid to assert herself. All this spelt *Silica*, and *Silica* in infrequent doses made a vast difference all round, even to her character!

Last winter after a good deal of domestic stress and strain, she developed a diffuse urticaria, all over her body which was very irritating, worse after washing, she also kept on complaining about feeling so cold right inside, her very bones, all her "innards" felt icy cold. One gave *Sulphur* 1m mainly on the symptom; urticaria worse for washing; and the skin eruption cleared up, and also much to my surprise, this icy cold feeling. On looking up *Sulphur* in Kent's *Repertory*, one saw *Sulphur* under the rubric, "icy cold feeling in the bones and inner parts," and I had always thought of *Sulphur* as a hot remedy, a remedy feeling the heat unduly. Verily *Sulphur* is a protean remedy, and one cannot get on without it.

This friend of mine, when the next autumn came along, started to complain again about the cold, how terribly cold it was, long before it was necessary, I thought. However, I promised her a remedy to warm her up, and she duly got *Silica xm.* High potencies do not work, some folks say; but believe it or not, a real cold spell with ground frost and cold northerly winds came along within twenty-four hours of her being given this dose of *Silica xm*; and I anxiously asked: "What about this cold weather?"— and to my surprise she replied that she had not felt it at all, even though she had been out visiting all day. It worked within twenty-four hours, yes, as quickly as all that! Suggestion maybe, but she does not take kindly to suggestion now, not since she has been put on *Silica*. No, no, she has quite a mind of her own. So you see, the right homœopathic medicine warms up a person, by acting on the heat-regulating mechanism of the body. Among other things it acts on the character and changes and alters it so that after some months you would hardly recognize her or him as the same individual.

My theme was prevention of disease by homœopathic means. Well, this lady's rheumatism has cleared up; her sore throats are a thing of the past; the lumbago and rheumatism of the leg and shoulder muscles never get a hold of her now; so Homœopathy has prevented the rheumatism from becoming chronic, has prevented heart disease, which follows so frequently after rheumatism. Is that not sufficient to show that the drugs applied according to the rule "like cures like"—act as preventives of disease?

Another curious action of the *Silica* in this particular case was its action upon the sweat glands. The perspiration under the arms was profuse, very strong and unpleasant all the year round, even in the winter. Various remedies had been applied to prevent this body odour with very little effect; but *Silica* also banished this unpleasant symptom in the correct homœopathic manner by curing from within, not by suppressing it and closing up the pores of the skin with local applications. Now *Silica* is not always the remedy to banish body odour : it might be any other remedy. You must remember that Homœopathy individualizes; each person must be taken as a single unit, and studied accordingly; and body odour is only one common symptom and not a very important one—except to the patient—from a prescriber's point of view. So body odour can be removed by any remedy which covers the important symptoms of the particular patient. And that is where the genius of the prescriber comes in, to discover these principal symptoms. And by uncovering these symptoms with the right remedy or sequence of right remedies—one can and does do true preventive work; one is enabled to prevent serious internal diseases. One can prevent heart disease, tuberculosis, etc., yea, even cancer can be prevented in the early days.

HOW TO CURE TONSILLITIS

THE seasonable indispositions, such as feverish chills and tonsillitis, attacked us very early in autumn 1933, very largely due to the hot summer and the prolonged drought. The streets were full of germ-laden dust, and the Public Health authorities were somewhat niggardly with watering the pavement. Result : outbreaks of "throats."

I speak feelingly, as I was a victim myself. It started with a feeling of extreme tiredness, headache, backache and heat plus chill and shivering on moving about. This suggested to me my old friend in acute troubles—*Nux vomica*. No good, the lassitude did not go, the chilliness disappeared; only a few symptoms were removed. It meant trying to find the whole picture of the acute remedy. I then noticed that my comfortable bed felt very hard, unusually so; my body was bruised, as if I had had a fall; my throat was aching, and the pain extended into my ears; I could not swallow hot tea, but liked cold orange juice. The tonsils were enormous, brilliantly red and studded with large yellow pustules, a typical *Phytolacca* throat. One dose of *Phytolacca* 30 was taken, and within twelve hours all the yellow pustules had disappeared, the temperature had dropped and, after repeating the *Phytolacca* every twelve hours, first in the 30th potency and later in the 200th, I was able to return to my duties after three days. No septic gargles, no nasty throat paints were required; it was a rapid, painless recovery.

I had quite a collection of acute cases of tonsillitis round about that time, and they all required different remedies. There was the young woman with the common symptoms of pain on swallowing, dryness of throat, enlarged purple tonsils, common symptoms to tonsillitis that is generally found in this disease. The other symptoms were individual ones and were used to find the correct remedies in each case. Her inflammation first started on the left side, and she could not bear warm drinks, could not swallow tea at all because of the choking it induced, saliva came away in long strings, and she felt worse during the night, woke up with clutching of the throat. *Lachesis* 30, four doses, settled her so that in twenty-four hours she could be pronounced well. I had another almost identical-looking sore throat, but it started on the right side, and the child liked warm drinks. I could get nothing else out of the child, but *Lycopodium* 6, four doses only, soon put the youngster right.

The worst case of acute tonsillitis I treated would not respond to the ordinary remedies; I tried *Phytolacca*, I tried *Mercury* because of the extremely dirty tongue, the extreme prostration and the offensive odour from the mouth, but neither would do, even though exhausting sweats were present as well. The patient was content to lie there and gave absolutely no help. "I have a sore throat and can't swallow, and you do the rest"; that was the attitude.

After looking at her for several days and trying various drugs, I saw *Mercurius protoiodatus* in her case. The right tonsil began by being inflamed, it spread to the left side which suggested *Lycopodium*, but she did not like warm drinks, cervical and parotid glands were tremendously swollen and tender. You could hardly see the throat on account of the accumulation of sticky mucous. The tongue was thickly coated at the base with thick yellowish fur. There was nausea at the sight of food, and a most penetrating offensive odour exuded from the patient. The abdomen was hard and painful to touch, and an almost complete stoppage of the bowels was present. Only tiny nodules were passed, and they only came away after great straining.

A doctor friend of hers saw her on a visit of compassion and considered she would be ill for at least a fortnight. Well, *Mercurius protoiodatus* 10m soon made a great difference. Almost overnight it all cleared up, throat better, spots on tonsils gone, voice not thick any more, tongue cleaner, offensive odour hardly noticeable. This derivative of *Mercury* did the trick, where the ordinary *Mercury* would not touch. Twenty-four hours after *Mercurius protoiodatus* had been given, the patient enjoyed a decent dinner and asked for more, and within a week she was back at her work. The *Mercurius protoiodatus* had to be repeated several times, three-hourly first, then three times a day, and after three days a dose was given, whenever the offensive odour reappeared.

This case reminds me of another I had some years ago, a quinsy. The patient lay like one dead, no reaction, could not swallow anything, only half conscious, the left side was mainly affected, there was a profuse flow of saliva, and the fauces were dark red. She seemed to be sinking from the acute toxæmia caused by the septic condition of the throat. I was very worried; should I call in a surgeon and have the abscess lanced? I could not really see down the throat, as the mouth could not be opened. There was such a search in the Materia Medica books for the right thing. Eventually I gave *Mercurius biniodatus* 10m, and do you know, within ten minutes—it seems unbelievable—the patient roused herself and said, "It has broken." She retched and brought up a large amount of foul-smelling pus. It just ran from her, and it was astounding to see how quickly all signs of tox-æmia disappeared. Death had been hovering very near; but the next day you would not have known her as the same person.

The other tonsillitis patient I saw was different again. She had agonizing pains in the head, could not bear the light, the throat was intensely red and swollen, the face was very red and hot, and she complained of her neck throbbing. *Belladonna* was the remedy here, and it cleared up the throat in the usual manner. So you see tonsillitis is a very common, everyday malady; but we have no specific. You may have to choose one of many drugs. As soon as you find the right medicine, the recovery is rapid.

No local treatment is required. Antiseptic paints, iodine gargles, hydrogen peroxide mouth washes, are unnecessary and, in fact, delay the cure. I should advise perhaps a tepid compress round the throat on the outside, if the pressure can be borne. It is comforting to many people. No solid food, while the temperature lasts, only fruit juices; orange juice and lemon juice are excellent. Absolutely the finest thing out for the throat that I know of, is pineapple. The tinned stuff is no good. It must be fresh juice. Pineapples contain certain digestive principles which clear up the mucous and the dirty tongue, membrane and septic patches on the tonsils, also it is very refreshing. After a day or two the juice becomes too astringent and it is better then to stop its ministration.

N.B. A tea gargle is helpful when fruit juices are not available. Add a cup of hot water to a teaspoonful of tea, boil for 15 minutes, adding more water when it is boiling away. This makes a weak solution of tannic acid. Put one tablespoonful of this solution in half a cup of hot water and gargle every four hours or so.

Tonsillitis is quite often fatal. Patients may linger for over a week in a state of almost complete coma, the weakness gets gradually worse and worse from the septic absorption and the inability to swallow. But, thanks to our wide choice of remedies, we can still bring the patient back—even from the very brink of the grave. Now for a short résumé of the principal drugs as they affect the throat :

Apis. Redness and swelling of throat with stinging and burning pains, ameliorated by cold, like an erysipelas of the throat. The tongue is swollen, also the uvula is swollen and puffed, and it resembles a water blister; direction of the swelling is from right to left. The patient desires a cold room, dislikes heat, such as the open fire. Fever without thirst.

N.B.—In some dangerous throat conditions the inflammation is almost painless.

Belladonna. Another right-sided remedy. Throat dry, bright red, burning, unable to swallow, especially fluids which may return through the nostrils, suggesting paralysis of muscles of deglutition. High fever present, patient intensely hot, face red and burning, blood-vessels throbbing, head throbbing, pain in throat extends to ear, is sensitive to pain, sensitive to light. *Belladonna* is very thirsty, craves for lemon juice; there is tenderness and enlargement of glands of neck at the beginning of a simple tonsillitis; it often aborts it.

Arsenic. Prostration is marked, burning throat, thirsty for frequently repeated sips of cold water—is most typical for *Arsenic* —restless and anxious, worse round about midnight or soon after.

Baptisia. Tonsils dusky, purplish red, great swelling, *painless* throat comes on very rapidly. Tongue swollen and offensive and purple, covered with thick brown fur down the centre, can swallow fluids, but not solids. General low state of patient which comes on very rapidly, extremely prostrated and rapidly sinks into stupor. Delirious and confused, seems to feel there are two of him.

Crotalus horridus. Left-sided throats with low form of blood poisoning. Bleeding from orifices of the body, body appears mottled, yellow and blue, gangrenous or diphtheritic throat, much swelling of glands, impossible to swallow liquids, throat slightly constricted. Low passive delirium, muttering and mumbling speech.

Lachesis. Left-sided or left to right. Sensation of fullness of neck, difficult breathing, choking on going to sleep or swallowing, aggravation of throat symptoms from warm drinks, unable to swallow, pain worse empty swallowing; purple throat.

Lac Caninum. Throat with alternating sides, right to left, and to right again, throat looks red and glazed and shiny with silver-grey deposit, pains relieved by swallowing cold or warm drinks.

Lycopodium. Right-sided remedy or right to left, relieved from swallowing warm drinks, opposite to Lachesis; and there is also no aggravation during sleep, and no constriction of throat. Pain extends into ear (as in *Belladonna, Hepar, Lachesis, Lac caninum, Phytolacca*).

Phytolacca. The vegetable Mercury is frequently indicated in sore throats, glands swollen, thick tenacious mucus, symptoms worse nights. Aching in all bones, body feels bruised and sore, bed feels hard. Mouth is fœtid, tongue coated, swallowing cold liquids relieves pain, warm drinks aggravate pain (*Lachesis*). Pain and stiffness in the cervical region.

Mercurius. Spongy throat, fullness and stiffness of neck, throat dry, swallowing is difficult, *Mercurial* odour marked. tongue thickly coated, takes imprint of teeth, sub-maxillary glands enlarged, dark red throat, acute prostration, weakness, offensive sweat, patient worse at night, trembling of limbs.

Mercurius protoiodatus. Strongly right-sided, remains on right side, tongue very thickly coated with yellow or light brown base, excessive secretion of tenacious mucus in the throat, which is difficult to move, especially in the morning, offensive fœtid odour, warm drinks aggravate pain (opposite *Lycopodium*), patient very languid and excessively tired, nausea at sight of food.

Mercurius biniodatus. Left to right, constant desire to hawk, a lump in throat, tenacious mucus, empty swallowing aggravates, glands swollen, fauces dark red, dreams troublesome, feels light-headed as if floating.

Hepar Sulphuris. Ulcers in throat, sensation of splinters or fish-bones in throat, pain extends to ear, on yawning and swallowing and turning the head, ameliorated by warm drinks (*Lycopodium*), patient feels very cold, particularly affected each time he goes out in dry cold winds, or cold east winds. Fever with sweating and a desire to be covered up; profuse perspiration, yet he wants several blankets over him; objects to draughts, open doors and windows.

Kali bichromicum. Has deep scooped-out ulcers on tonsils, the saliva is sticky and stringy.

Since writing the above one has recalled several other adventures with tonsillitis. To me sore throat is like an undesirable neighbour, always near at hand or lurking around the corner when least wanted. The most exciting personal encounter one had was during a three months' clinical clerkship in a Continental mental hospital. The authorities believed in keeping their patients warm and coddled them unduly; open windows were frowned upon, and one's duties kept one indoors. One day I found myself laid out, delirious and with a rapidly forming quinsy. The head physician visited me four times a day as he was so worried, temperature of 104 degrees, he murmured and shook his head. He ordered salicylates and throat compresses. One recalls the total disregard of his instructions, the nursing attention was just nil, one was severely left alone. After thirty-six hours of this, my professional pride and love of life roused me up to make an effort to help myself. So one of the patients on parole was sent out surreptitiously and smuggled in some *Belladonna 3x* and *Mercurius dulcis 3x*, which I took alternately three-hourly after the good old fashion of the earlier Homœopaths. I staggered into the bathroom, I remember, and damping bathtowels, applied a rough and ready wet compress round back and chest. To the visiting doctor's great surprise, the temperature was down next morning, and the quinsy resolving fast. He could not make it out at all and prophesied I should be in bed over Easter, which was five days ahead. I smiled feebly, and two days later he had to give permission to get up, as I was so well and clamouring to be up. One also recalls his order to the Steward's department to supply two bottles of malt beer as a daily tonic, which the attendant was delighted to consume in my stead. I was impressed by the quick results of the homœopathic remedies. One day nearly dead, and the next day all danger past and the quick recovery! All this was put down by the allopathic physician to my strong constitution. After this adventure, one hastened to shake the dust of that unpleasant institution off one's feet, and left it for other shores, where fresh air, and plenty of it, was the order of the day.

Recently I had another "do" with tonsillitis, quite out of the blue again it came, temperature, a thickly coated tongue, weariness, bruised backache and sore feeling all over the body : difficulty of swallowing at the root of the tongue and the big yellow pustules on the swollen left tonsil. No desire for food, hot drinks impossible to swallow, but cold orange juice was most agreeable : *Phytolacca*, of course. As it was absolutely essential I should be back at work in twenty-four hours, I took it two-hourly in the 30th potency. As a rule, one likes to experiment on oneself and see how long one dose of the remedy will act and waits until the action is played out. Within twenty-four hours I was perfectly all right and was able to give an hour's lecture, without my throat giving out or a return of the old enemy : I took *Phytolacca* three times a day for another two days, and then no more. No other remedy was needed, as I felt perfectly fit and well.

After acute remedies or short acting remedies in an acute ill-ness, specially after acute tonsillitis, or septic throats, the consti-tutional remedy is usually required, and unless there are strong indications for any particular remedy the best one to give for tiredness, weakness, hot flushes on the slightest exertion, when moving in bed or talking on the telephone or thinking of work, is our great friend in need—*Sulphur*, which removes the damp heat and uncomfortable tiredness and dislike for work in a very short time. Always remember, therefore, *Sulphur* in debility after tonsillitis.

One just recalls a doctor friend who had several bouts of septic tonsillitis, while our orbits crossed. She was fond of dosing herself with salicylates and using the strongest antiseptic gargles, such as chlorine gargles alternating with hydrogen peroxide, and later taking quinine tonics to pull herself into shape again. Dura-tion of illness and off-duty time ten days! and under homœo-pathic treatment twenty-four to seventy-two hours!

Common sense would tell one that Homœopathy was a better proposition for a person with any kind of sore throat than the orthodox way of treating it. Why not try it?

Rheumatic sore throat is very common in this damp maritime climate of ours. The usual suggestion for it is : excision of the tonsils; unfortunately this does not prevent further attacks of painful swollen throats, as one has proved to one's satisfaction many times. The condition recurs again and again, and is rather worse than it was before the removal of the tonsils. You see, as we Homœopaths say, the disease product has been removed, but not the cause; find the cause and the disease will disappear; and the cause can be treated and removed by Homœopathy so easily and painlessly. I have a friend who had been suffering from rheu-matism of the throat for years, tonsils were duly removed, and the throats went gaily on, crippling her and incapacitating her many times. They usually came in wet weather (*Calcarea, Dulc.,*

Hep., Rhus tox.); there was pain on swallowing food and on empty swallowing, warmth in general removed it (*Hep., Rhus tox.*), there was stiffness of the throat (*Rhus tox.*) and œdematous swelling of the throat, and a sensation, as if the throat was all swollen up and closed, choking sensation on swallowing liquids and a grasping pain, as if something was being torn out of the throat. *Rhus tox.* has all these symptoms, and *Rhus tox.* 6, given in repeated doses, cured this throat very rapidly, and at the slightest return of these symptoms a dose or two suffices to abort an attack; and for ten years or so this enthusiastic believer in Homœopathy—has she not proved in herself how marvellously it works?—has never had a day's illness or stayed away from work.

It is a joy to treat acute diseases with homœopathic remedies, they respond so quickly; and it is a pity that doctors in general, and the public do not know more about it. Aspirin, and the various other brands of it, do not work anything like as well, chloride of potash gargles and internal medication are much slower in action, and very disagreeable to take. I tried chloride of potash on myself, while a house surgeon, on the recommendation of my chief, but gave it up very soon for the pleasant, more efficacious sugar pills.

In recurrent attacks of tonsillitis and septic throats each acute attack should be treated by the indicated acute remedy; but the acute remedy is only short acting, it requires the constitutional remedy to prevent a recurrence; there one has a variety of remedies to choose from. Again, it might be *Sulphur* or *Calcarea* or *Baryta carb.* or *Silica* or *Lycopodium* or *Phos.* or any other, as indicated by the symptoms of the individual. One should never generalize, and again, as I have said again and again, there are no specifics, and each individual has to be studied, until the correct remedy is found, and enlarged septic tonsils will disappear with the remedy, if you give it time. Very few tonsil operations are necessary and should be avoided as much as possible. Build up the patient first with his or her constitutional remedy, and during the process of building up, even septic tonsils have been known to disappear; if the tonsils become fibrosed and refuse to disappear entirely, that is the time to operate; the enlarged tonsils are just foreign bodies. Then what a saving of hospital beds this would mean, as nearly 25 per cent. of all operations are tonsil operations.

EARACHE

EARACHE, like all bone pains, is described by its sufferers as being maddening or excruciating in nature. The technical term is acute middle-ear disease, it follows on after such acute diseases as influenza, measles, scarlet fever, etc., or even ordinary tonsillitis or exposure to draughts and strong winds. A common cause nowadays is in motorists: people sitting in saloon cars being driven along at speeds of thirty to forty or more miles an hour, all the windows closed except the driver's and a small ventilating opening in the roof; thus the driver and the passenger in the front are sitting in a direct current of cold air which strikes the back of the neck and the ear. Consequence: earache, and frequently a mastoid operation.

How often does one hear these days of mastoid trouble in the young well-to-do motoring fraternity! And yet how easily could incision of the drum, and the more serious mastoid operation, be avoided, if Homœopathy were used for the early stages of middle-ear disease.

A middle-aged woman after a motoring week-end was seen, complaining of pain in left ear, fullness, dullness and muffled sensation in front of ear; touch and pressure made the pain worse. The history of pain after exposure to cold air led me to prescribe *Merc. bin.* 6 for this lady with very happy results. Not only did the bulging inflamed eardrum return to normal, but also a nasal polypus which was discovered at the same time and of which the patient had not the slightest idea, dried up and disappeared after a month's treatment, and the nasal catarrh which had bothered her for months cleared up as well. She talked of going to an ear specialist and having an operation for the polypus, but when the earache disappeared, she decided to wait until after the summer holiday which was just due; and when she was seen again, there wasn't any polypus left, and surgery was superfluous. I don't know that she was particularly grateful: people nowadays do like boasting of all the operations they have had, and I shrewdly suspect that she thought in her own mind I had made a mistake in finding a nasal polypus the first time.

Incidentally, it reminds me of another incident which had happened many years ago in my childhood days. There was a great commotion in the nursery one morning : the little sister had been delirious all night with flaming hot cheeks and acute ear-ache. The anxious mother rushed her off at once to the best known professor of ear diseases in the local University town, who shook his head and talked learnedly of incising the drum. The honoured parent, who was a staunch Homœopath, would not hear of it, but begged for twenty-four hours' grace. Reluctantly she was allowed to take the child home, with all kinds of dire threats. Undeterred by all this, she started giving *Belladonna* 3x in watery solution every half-hour, and when the professor saw the little patient twenty-four hours later he was sorely puzzled as to what had happened to the inflamed drum; he looked at the ear, then at his notes, and again peered into the ear. "Mrs. ——, are you sure this is the same child I saw yesterday?" He called his assistant, they came to the conclusion that something extra-ordinary, something they had never seen before, had happened —an inflamed ear had resolved without operative interference ! Mother was jubilant, and never failed to tell this tale against the famous surgeon, where Homœopathy had triumphed and carried the day.

This incident made a deep impression, and since that day I have saved many people from incision of the drum. *Belladonna* is not always the remedy, nor is *Merc. biniodide*. It depends on the symptoms which are present, such as the nature of the pain, the direction, the ameliorations and aggravations of the local seat of trouble.

We were called one evening to a little fair-haired boy, almost beside himself with pain in the ear; he was fretful and whiny, wanted to be made a fuss of; the pain came on in fits and shot right down to the teeth in the lower jaw. All these details pointed to *Pulsatilla*, and a few doses of *Puls.* high cleared up the inflamed drum in less than twenty-four hours. For two or three years afterwards he had a recurrence of this trouble which always came on after he got his feet wet, another *Puls.* symptom. It is now several years since his last attack, and one knows, should there be a recurrence, *Puls.* will again help, as sure as anything.

Another case occurred in a young student after German measles. She presented the typical *Pulsatilla* symptoms, and it cleared up as suddenly as it came after a few doses, without leaving any deafness behind or any other symptoms of eustachian catarrh. Chronic deafness is the usual sequel after otitis media in German measles, as treated by orthodox methods!

Belladonna, Pulsatilla, Merc. bin. are common remedies in cases of acute earache; but other drugs may be required, and one has to study one's Materia Medica carefully to find the right remedy.

Once a boy was brought in for earache during the teething period. He was shrieking the place down, so spiteful, nothing was right for him; he wanted to be carried about; he hit his mother; one side of his face was red and the other pale; he could not speak yet, but there was no need to ask many questions: the remedy stared one in the face; it was *Chamomilla*, and the next time this child was seen, there was not a better behaved child in creation, a perfect angel, and his earache had gone without an operation.

Much about the same time another infant, about fourteen months old, was seen with almost identical symptoms. He was irritable and fretful, did not want to be touched, screamed when the back of the ear was touched; but the face was pale and he rolled his head. I diagnosed otitis media, and examination with an ear speculum confirmed it. The remedy was *Cina*, in this case; but unfortunately it was not in stock and, before it could be procured, the mother had become too worried and worked up and had rushed the child off the same day to a local hospital, where an operation was performed twenty-four hours later, first an incision of the drum, later a complete mastoid, and three or four days later the child was in the *post mortem* room. One could not blame the mother: she did what she thought best under the circumstances.

A very similar case was seen very shortly afterwards. The child showed the same rolling of the head, the same irritability and sensitiveness to touch; did not want anybody to come near him, was constantly picking his nose. The mother, of course, thought it was worms and had considered giving him a worm cake which is largely made up of santonin; the source, as John H. Clarke puts it, of our homœopathic *Cina*. I dissuaded the mother, as the santonin would have made the condition much worse; but I knew that the homœopathic *Santonin* given in minutest subdivision and dilution would certainly cure here, as the child during his illness showed the very same symptoms, as were brought out by the healthy provers, when they took repeated doses and noted the effects produced on themselves. These signs and symptoms I repeat again were : this normally affectionate child refused to be touched or caressed; tossed about in bed and rolled his head; the face was pallid with a white line round the mouth, gritted his teeth and picked his nose; the temperature was 101°, the drum of the ear was bulging and red. How difficult it was to examine it! *Cina* 30 four-hourly quickly altered this serious state of affairs, and three days later once again we had a bright, affectionate child, with a sound eardrum and no brain complications.

"Coincidence," you say; but if one gets case after case showing symptoms which a homœopathic doctor recognizes as being found under a certain remedy, and when he applies that remedy, and the particular pathological disease clears up immediately, surely a logical mind would ascribe the cure to the remedy, the medicine given, and not to some mythical coincidence. But some folks are difficult to convince and will wriggle out of any argument, if it does not suit them to believe.

Now still another case in a baby, before I quote some cases of earache in adults.

In one way children are difficult to treat, as you have to depend entirely on your powers of observation; you cannot ask any questions as regards the nature, the seat, and the character and directions of the pain. On the other hand, their objective signs and symptoms are clearer, not disguised or hidden by crude drugs and large doses of medicines taken in the past.

This baby was eight months old and just passing through its difficult period of dentition : breast fed, with a good careful mother, a happy, contented mortal, always cooing and laughing. Suddenly it all changed, the face became scarlet and felt very hot to the touch; the temperature was 102°, and he was delirious during the night, constantly shrieking with piercing shrieks, the throat was intensely red, and the left eardrum was red and bulging. "Did I incise its eardrum?" I should have, according to recognized and orthodox teaching. I depended on the homœopathic scalpel, which in this case was *Belladonna*. The district nurse was sent in to watch the case, and if necessary, send it to hospital; but again the simple remedy conquered the foul disease; the temperature went down to 99° the next morning and never went up again, and the child recovered as quickly as it was stricken down.

In the early days of practice in cases of this nature, earache with red congested drums and tenderness over the mastoid, I frequently went to a case with fear and trembling on the second visit, gas bag and ear instruments, fine scalpels, etc., all at hand in case of need, but it was never necessary. I never had to do this small, delicate operation which every practitioner should be able to do, as text-books tell you, to prevent the more serious extension of the disease into the mastoid cavity, which may mean more trouble, and months and months of discharging ears, deafness and perhaps death.

How much easier it all is, to procure a resolution of an inflamed middle ear by a few doses of the indicated remedy. Perhaps it is too easy, and on the whole not spectacular enough! One would miss the glamour and ritual of the whole surgical procedure, the bustling nurse, the cheerful anæsthetist with his bagful of sweet-smelling mystery, and the important Jove-like surgeon who holds death and life in his glistening instruments and his dexterous hands. All glory to the clever mechanician when he is needed; but if Homœopathy was known and properly applied, the surgeon would once more occupy the secondary place of importance, once held in the old days of the barber surgeon.

Speaking of surgeons and specially aural surgeons, I remember a very puzzled colleague, a specialist, who, when told that a nurse was suffering from acute middle-ear disease with deafness, acute earache and faceache, enlarged glands of the neck and tonsillitis, warned the said nurse, how serious such a condition was and offered to do all he could for her in using his influence getting her into hospital and having her operated on. She refused his very kind offer and stuck to Homœopathy. A couple of weeks later this self-same aurist was more than surprised to see the nurse back at work, well and blooming—earache gone, faceache and sore throat gone, no discharging ears and no deafness and no noises in the head!

"What treatment did you have," he asked, "to get well so quickly; two weeks ago, you were very ill, and now you are recovered! You say, you had medicine, nothing else, no specific ear treatment. Astonishing, you must have a wonderful constitution."

I could have told him, that this rapid cure was due to *Bella-donna*, as she had *Belladonna* symptoms; the sudden rapid onset, the high temperature, the throbbing pulsations in the head, all caused by exposure to cold wind and chill of the head; wearing a nurse's cap all day, and going out to a theatre minus a head covering at night.

As it happened, she had had one or two minor attacks during the previous three months, and the ear surgeons—there were three at the aural clinic she worked at—talked of advising a three-months rest and change for her, to clear up this tendency to otitis media.

One saw, that *Belladonna* did not hold the case; it did not prevent a recurrence, it was not deep-acting enough; so in the last and third most serious attack, after relieving the acute pain with *Belladonna*, one went on and gave *Merc. bin.* and *Merc. bin.* 4th centesimal dilution, given night and morning for a fort-night, cleared up the ear and also the tendency to earache with each change in the weather.

As I said, the ear specialist was astonished, but he put it down to constitution or a mere happy fluke.

Poor man, he could do with a little Homœopathy himself, he is frightened of a bit of wind or draught, always cossets himself, always has a cold and cough, always afraid of broncho-pneu-monia to which he is subject. And all the advice he could give the sister was "be careful of colds and draughts"—but how? He did not say "by wrapping up", it did not prevent colds in his own case.

Another nurse had suffered from pain and deafness in the right ear; a fullness and numbness and muffled feeling of the ear and right side of face which had persisted for about three weeks.

The general practitioner told her it was due to the change and gave her valerian and bromide, with no result. She was getting deafer every day, and the numbness of the face grew worse; every breath of cold wind made the faceache worse; she could not stoop because of the feeling in the ear. She also was given *Merc. biniodide* 6 twice a day, and on account of the complete deafness of the right ear due to eustachian catarrh following an acute middle-ear disease, she was politzerized and had to have a eustachian catheter passed to open the closed passages leading to the ear. She required a month's treatment and was then discharged without a trace of deafness.

Just at that time, I had a run of ear cases, all showing *Merc. bin.* symptoms: left-sided earache caused by cold air, dullness and numbness of left side of face with feeling of internal heat of vertex, and side affected: deafness after getting warm, giddiness which made it impossible to stoop; one often notices in the course of the years that a certain remedy seems to be more in the running during a certain period, and then a few months later the same disease—the same pathological entity requires a totally different remedy or set of remedies to cure it; the picture of the current epidemic always changes; and one has to study each manifestation of an acute illness afresh. I can just recall two nurses, two teachers, one headmaster and a woman doctor all with earache, and all yielding to *Merc. bin.*

But enough of *Merc. biniodide,* or you will run away with the idea, which is the last thing I wish for, that this is a specific for earache; and there "ain't such a thing" as specifics for a disease in Homœopathy. Let me illustrate this:

Some fifteen years ago I was called to a midwife who was laid low with a high temperature, ulcerated throat, and acute earache on the right side. I gave *Belladonna*, with the result that the next day the pain in the right ear had gone, the drum had lost its ominous redness, and the patient was on the mend, I thought. Unfortunately I crowed too soon, the next day exactly the same trouble reappeared, but this time in the left ear, the temperature went up, the left drum was red and swollen, and so on. Once again I thought, I should need to call in surgery to my aid, but I remembered the *Lycopodium* symptom: "disease going from right to left," and on that gave *Lycopodium.*

I had another case almost identical, at that time, in the next street, and so they both got *Lycopodium.* The next day I went along with gas bag and other necessaries for incising the drums of the two patients, and lo! they had both cleared up, temperature was down, and both were pleased. Again I was triumphant too early. In one of the cases *Lyc.* proved all efficient, and no further remedy was required for curing the acute ear; but in the case of the midwife I was confronted once again with a rise of temperature to 101° on the next visit, recrudescence of the acute earache in the right ear, the right tonsil was swollen and glazed and shiny, and the left ear was quite normal. I was not beaten, however, Homœopathy did not fail me. I remembered that *Lac. caninum* has this symptom, as Kent puts it: complaints, regardless of kind or quality, change sides; and *Lac. caninum* 900, four-hourly, effected the almost impossible. This time the drum went back to normal, the tonsil cleared up, and there was no return of any inflammation, and no incision of the drum was required, no deafness followed and there was no extension of the disease to the mastoid. A most satisfactory result to the patient.

Now still another case, and still another remedy. This was a lady who had a mastoid operation on her left ear many, many years ago, but still gets acute earache or faceache off and on. She had a particularly severe "go" a few weeks ago, with the following details: left-sided, very acute cutting, stitching pains over ear, shooting down into lower jaw and up to crown of head, very bad during daytime, much easier during night, any motion, stooping, etc., was unbearable, could not bite or chew even the softest of foods. Warmth relieved. She was very gloomy and depressed and very disinclined to move or work, most unlike her normal busy self. She was naturally very agitated about the mastoid inflammation recurring again. After two or three days of intense suffering she was given *Spigelia* 30 three-hourly, which speedily removed all pain and suffering. It had another curious sequel: a large lump of hard, inspissated earwax was found lying the next morning on the piece of cotton wool which she had put in her ear to keep out the cold air. One argues from this: that the piece of wax was pressing on the superficial nerves in the ear and causing the acute neuralgia; once the pressure of the wax was removed, the pain went. Was it a coincidence that a piece of hard wax which was lying deep down in the cavity suddenly loosened on its own? Or was it due to the action of the *Spigelia* which was given twelve hours previously? You can believe what you like. This lady had bouts of pains several times for two years increasing in intensity, subsiding each time without specific treatment, until it reached its climax. Since the *Spigelia* was given, all discomfort and pain has gone.

Earache during menopause is almost always relieved by *Gels*. The pain comes on after exposure to cold air and is of congestive nature; the ear feels hot and full, the lobe of the ear is red and burning, and the extremities feel cold. There is giddiness, and weight and tiredness of limbs. When you give *Gels*. for earache or faceache of this nature, it will disappear quickly; and as pain is relieved, the patient has to pass large quantities of clear, watery urine.

Glonoin is sometimes needed in these menopausal cases of congestive headaches and earaches, violent pulsations and throbbing in ear and head, pain easier in the open air, worse from warmth and lying down, has to sit bolstered up in bed, cold applications relieve. I know a lady who is always quickly improved from the rushing pains in her ears by a few doses of *Glonoin*. She can neither stand the heat nor the sun, and is always seen walking about with a large sunshade and an old-fashioned large shady hat.

There is one type of earache which requires *Hepar sulph.*, one variety of subacute otitis media, where the drum is very near rupturing, the pain is so acute and patient is nearly driven mad with it. Cold air, cold draught and open air make it worse, the pain is unbearable at night, and the only thing that relieves it, is wrapping up the ear and head with a warm shawl. In this it resembles *Chamomilla*, only a *Chamomilla* patient is even more spiteful, gives way to violent frenzy and outbursts of anger. The *Hepar* individual is more likely to faint with the acuteness of the pain.

I nearly forgot *Ferrum Phos.* in acute otitis media. There was a girl of 12 years of age who in two years had at least six attacks of acute earache, her drum had been incised two or three times. Earache aggravated by cold air, skin hot and dry, red cheeks, half-open eyelids, a modified *Belladonna* case; nose bleeding with each attack. *Ferrum Phos.* 12 as soon as an attack started would abort it in 12-24 hours. I watched her for three years; and occasional doses of this remedy always helped her each time. When seen last, she had had no attacks for 18 months.

Capsicum is an important remedy for threatened mastoid abscess. Earache worse at night, redness and flush over the mastoid process, cheeks are red and cold. I have averted a mastoid operation on several occasions by this remedy, which has a peculiar specific action on the bones of the internal ear and the mastoid process.

I have only considered a few of the more ordinary medicines required to relieve earache, in different individuals. I must repeat again, there are no specifics in Homœopathy, you must study each case individually, take the particulars carefully, observe all the details, and then you will be successful in preventing serious troubles, long-standing invalidism which is the result of "badly treated earache." At a future date I hope to discuss chronic ear discharge and its successful homœopathic treatment.

DIFFICULT CHILDREN

EARLY one Sunday morning the landlady of a superior boarding house in the West End was awakened by the insistent ringing of the house telephone. The voice on the other end of the wire which she recognized as that of one of her most troublesome lady boarders, insisted that Dr. —— must be sent for at once, as she was feeling very ill. The proprietress not recognizing the name, asked who he was and got the reply: "Don't you remember, he was the doctor I read about in the library book last week? It is urgent, I like the sound of his name, I must have him."

It was pointed out to her that this was a fictitious name, and the doctor did not exist, but this did not avail at all. Contradiction made Miss B., the boarder, only more and more angry and to pacify her, the telephone book was produced, and a doctor with a somewhat similar name was found. That was the reason why an astonished surgeon got an early summons to attend this lady. When he arrived at the house and knocked at this lady's door, to his surprise he was greeted by his patient brandishing a poker and threatening to do him in. He was a surgeon familiar with people's insides, but not with the crooked workings of a diseased mind. He fled for his life and hastily sprinted into the lady's bedroom and locked the door between them, while the patient continued to rave and break up the furniture and ornaments. He called out of the window to attract the attention of a passer-by—a rarity in a quiet square on Sunday morning. Eventually he managed to get a policeman so that he could be released from his ignominious position, and the poor demented lady was secured and sent off to a private home, where they had all the facilities to deal with people suffering from brain-storms. One heard that this lady, now quite elderly, had been afflicted from early childhood days with similar attacks of rage and temper, which used to come on without any warning. When out with her nurse she would suddenly throw herself down in the street, kick her legs, shout and scream, had to be held down and was frequently carried home by a policeman or in a cab, a fighting, screaming fury. There was no repression in her case, she was allowed to carry on and please herself. Her parents, one presumes, sought medical advice, and all they were told was, she would outgrow it! She certainly never did. As a young lady in late Victorian days, she used to upset the decorous company at luncheon or dinner with her storms and tempers, and so she had to be sent in the end to an asylum for restraint! She would have saved her parents, herself and her neighbours much anxiety, if she had been treated as a child by Homœopathy. This is not an idle or exaggerated statement.

Let me quote similar cases I have come across, who have been successfully dealt with. The second child of superior working-class people was a sullen, bad-tempered mite, even at a year old. Never a smile out of her; she would not play with anybody, she gave vent to terrible storms of temper, kicking and howling, and nobody, not even her father, could control her. She would not do anything she was told—the older she grew, the worse her tempers became. I tried to coax her, and give advice to her parents, but neither soft words, nor harshness made any difference. She remained just a "difficult child," her older brother, a sweet-tempered, happy boy tried to reason with her; but little Christine would have none of it and continued in her evil ways. This was years ago, and I bethought myself of similar cases I had read of in the Materia Medica books, and suggested to the mother, if she was willing, I should cure her girl of her tempers. She was only too glad, and so it came about that little Christine was given *Tuberculinum* 30 : several weekly doses. The first dose already made a difference and after a few weeks, the once sulky, bad-tempered child began to smile instead of frowning and turning her head away or even lashing out with her feet. She grew into a good-natured, happy child, and at the slightest return of temper she would get another dose of *Tuberculinum*. Her mother and father were always extremely grateful, and she used to say with tears in her eyes how wonderful those little powders were which turned her naughty girl into a happy, obedient one. One watched this little girl for several years until her parents left the neighbourhood, and there had been no need for "repetition of the dose" for many moons. The old Adam had been conquered.

Another case : One day at the Clinic, one heard a great commotion going on in the next room, much noisy altercation, at last the door opened and in came a young Englishwoman, trying hard to bring her twin girls in to see me. They were not yet two years of age, but they were as determined as their mother, that they had no wish to come and see the doctor in the white coat. They were Anglo-Chinese girls, with pretty slit almond eyes, and pink cheeks on an olive foundation, and had just returned from Carshalton Hospital after several months' treatment for severe rickets. Children of mixed races, Anglo-Chinese or Anglo-Negroid parentage do not stand our climate very well, even though they are born here, their bones seem very soft and bend easily and the worst rickets I have seen in latter years have been in children of a negro, or Chinese father and English mother. At Carshalton, as many such pretty children, they had been very much petted by the nurses and thoroughly spoilt, and now they were quite out of hand. The mother dragged one way with one child in each hand, and the little girls dragged another way, noisily protesting, and the next thing I saw, both children were on the floor with their legs in the air, kicking and screaming, nobody could make themselves heard above this din. It was impossible to do anything that day with these two minxes. I procured some *Tuberculinum* 30, and put it on their tongues, while each child was bellowing loudly. It was somewhat of a feat to get past those furiously kicking legs; the hospital had apparently made the nether extremities strong and capable of inflicting damage.

The children were carried out in the end by a hot mother with many apologies and planked into the pram. A week passed, the door opened and in came two tiny mites, hand-in-hand, allowing themselves to be examined without a murmur, my little demons of the week before! softened by *Tuberculinum*. They became quite reformed characters, we never had any more such exhibitions, though they were given a course of *Tuberculinum* for several months; they remained imps of mischief, who loved smearing brooms with jam, pulling the tablecloth off again as soon as it was set for dinner, going into the cupboards and mixing the sugar and the soap flakes and salt all together. They were always up to something new, but their tempers were *cured*. This mother was very prolific and produced a child every year. I think we dealt with five or six of her offspring and the interesting point was: that each child at about 18 months developed those terrific tempers, but they were one and all settled with a few doses of *Tuberculinum*. No stick was needed, no prolonged treatment and observation at child guidance clinics; they just calmed down after *Tuberculinum*.

It is sometimes very difficult to get the fond mothers to acknowledge that their children, specially their boys, are suffering from attacks of violent rage; one often has to wait, until one sees a child in an attack. There was a mother I remember, she had a boy after nearly sixteen years interval, he was made much of naturally, and when he was four, he became almost unmanageable; he appeared to be quiet and saint-like, just looking at you quite knowingly, while the mother told of these scenes. He appeared quite rational and she would take him out into the park, he would play for a while and then suddenly, for no apparent reason, he would go off into one of his tantrums, howl and scream and throw himself on the ground and make an exhibition of her. The neighbours would blame her for being cruel to him, when she had done nothing to him. She would take him to the local welfare centre or hospital, and the same thing would happen there: screams and kicking of feet and hitting the mother, so the mother was reduced to tears in her helplessness and could not take him anywhere with her. He was a thin, undersized child with fair hair, blue sclerotics, red lips, strawberry tongue and profuse growth of hair between the shoulder blades along the spine. She did not know what to do with him, he was a trouble and great anxiety to her. He had the physical characteristics of *Tuberculinum*, as just described, as well as the mental symptoms of uncontrollable rage. I consoled the mother as well as I could, assuring her that her boy could be cured, and needless to say with a few infrequent doses of *Tuberculinum*, along with bi-weekly sittings of ultra-violet rays, we succeeded in turning the boy into a normal tempered, happy individual. The symptoms that first drew attention to this remedy are found in Allen's *Materia Medica* as follows:

"Does not like to be disturbed by people; trembling of hands.

"Felt positively ugly; personal aversion almost became a mania.

"Trifles produced intense irritation and could not be shaken off.

"Very irritable, wanted to fight, no hesitancy in throwing anything at any one, even without a cause."

There was another boy who used to throw himself under the table, kick hard with his feet and shriek and shriek and many times upset the table with all the crockery on it. *Tuberculinum* rapidly put an end to these brain-storms.

Another symptom that always makes me give *Tuberculinum* to a young child is this : I offer the baby over a year old, an unmedicated tablet of sugar, if the child refuses to take it even though you coax it and say, "Have a sweet," and when you put the sweet on the child's tongue he immediately becomes obstreperous, refuses to swallow it and spits it out; his mother tries him and he clenches his teeth, and if she manages to push the sweet in, he still ejects it violently, one is pretty certain that *Tuberculinum* is the remedy and that after a few doses, the child will become lamblike and lose the tendency to these storms.

In the last ten years one has had many children from one to five years and over, with symptoms like those mentioned, and *Tuberculinum* 30 invariably helped. These fits of anger might come on with the teething, sometimes it might be a little later. A history of tuberculosis in some member of the family could not always be obtained, but one has a shrewd suspicion that there is a tubercular tendency in that family. The poorer classes do not know much about members of their family, of even a generation back; some prefer to lie and will not tell you the truth. But in quite a goodly percentage I have discovered that there has been tuberculosis in the family. These children with sudden brainstorms who react so well to *Tuberculinum* may require other medicines later on; but for a time they will do well on this remedy, and some seem to require nothing but *Tub.* to turn them into strong, healthy children with a normal amount of naughtiness, which is easily controllable.

A girl of 9 or 10 was brought to me two years ago with the history of snoring at night, and the mother wanted to know whether she had enlarged tonsils and adenoids; she had taken her to four different throat clinics, and none of the surgeons had been able to persuade her to open her mouth for examination. I found her a badly-nourished girl; everything went off swimmingly, we were good friends, until I asked her to let me look at her mouth. She was seized with unreasoning terror, would not be quietened, shrieked and yelled, it took four adults to hold her;

she subsided on the floor, taking two of the adults with her, tables and chairs flew in every direction, her eyes became glassy, she screamed, "I'll kill you, I'll kill you." I hastily removed myself outside the radius of those thrashing legs and sent for some *Tuberculinum* 30. It was a terrible struggle to make her take the tablet. The first tablet was ejected with great force and landed on the window sill; the second disappeared and was spat out and disappeared into another corner; the third was firmly placed inside the mouth and the nose and mouth were finally closed, so that eventually she had to swallow it. She was exhausted, and so were we all; and we thankfully saw the back of her.

The next week she returned, she made no murmur at my placing the spatula inside her mouth and let me examine her, and I hardly recognized her as the same spitting fury of a wild cat of the week before. As she had diseased septic tonsils which were foreign bodies and no good to her, she was recommended for operation. One heard later, she did not play up again as she did previous to the dose of *Tuberculinum* : so add this symptom to the list mentioned above.

"Unreasoning terror in a child at a medical examination or with strangers—*Tuberculinum*."

Now another difficult child with slightly different symptoms who was again cured by *Tuberculinum*, though I used a different preparation, namely Koch's *Tuberculinum*. There are different Tuberculins on the market; but they all act on the "tuberculinum" child, and one uses them at random.

This girl, $5\frac{1}{2}$ years old, was brought in September, 1936, with the following history : delicate child, "night screaming" as an infant, showed signs of an enlarged gland in the neck early in 1934. Taken to hospital, where her gland was operated on and also a culminating mastoid infection required an emergency operation. Since the operation she had developed frequent recurrent feverish attacks about every six weeks with vomiting; typical attacks of acidosis; the mastoid wound had never healed up, at the base an area nearly one inch across was still visible with a sinus leading down to the deeper tissue of the ear. The scar over the cervical gland looked unhealthy and showed typical puckering. She was on a rigid diet, non-fat, with skimmed milk, steamed vegetables, brown bread, potato, lettuce, cereal pudding with prune juice; and still the recurrent vomiting attacks persisted.

Family history: the mother had been in Margate as a young woman for six months for early pre-tubercular debility.

Psychologically the child was distinctly difficult, extremely excitable, argumentative, contrary, contradicting the whole time. "A 'no child' " with a vengeance; did always the opposite to what she was asked to do, restless, fidgety. While in my room, she played with the blind until she broke it, even though her mother begged her not to; went to all my drawers, picked things out of them, threw them about, looked at picture books for a minute, threw them aside—refused to be examined, refused to have her clothes off, had to be coaxed and argued with, was extremely obstinate, was said to be affectionate and liked sympathy, jumped about a lot, squeaking and making a noise even while I was talking to her mother. She was a sallow, dark, thin child—always hungry and yet never growing fat; very difficult in hospital, great many scenes while her wounds were being dressed after the operations, very prudish, disliked bathing costumes, impatient, great fear of dogs; weight 2 st. 10 lbs. *Tuberculinum* Koch 30 was prescribed, and soon made a great difference.

A month later she had gained a pound in weight, had had no sick headaches, no feverish attacks, *no vomiting on a normal diet*; the mastoid wound had healed over for the first time in $2\frac{1}{2}$ years—the night sweats had disappeared; though still hot when excited or running about; heavy odour about her bedroom from her body in the morning after a night's sleep; constipation—an old symptom—much improved.

December 8th, 1936. Not so excited, used to eat no breakfast before a journey, but now has a good meal. My secretary remarked how much quieter she was, while sitting in the waiting room; she used to upset and worry and annoy the other people, always in and out of the room, "an impossible child she was at first" she exclaimed; now the girl would sit and look at books for quite a long time and not disturb anybody.

Gained 6 lbs. in weight since September on a normal diet, no catarrh, no vomiting, no feverish attacks, a strong sound scar over the mastoid; continued *Tuberculinum* Koch 1m.

February 2nd, 1937. Gained $9\frac{1}{2}$ lbs. since September, 1936, not so excitable, no feverish chills now, even though she had a cold during the middle of December.

March 29th, 1937. Very constipated, put on bran and Agar Agar—no offensive perspiration now; very well otherwise, gained in weight, not afraid of the dark or dogs now; much quieter and not so argumentative.

June 18th, 1937. Frequent colds during spring, but no pyrexia, no vomiting, no night sweats, feels cold very much, feet sweat, catches colds from being overheated. Still contrary, fearful, bursts into tears for nothing; has not been well since her vaccination. The disease picture is changing from *Tuberculinum* and the complementary remedy *Silica* 30 was now given for footsweat, fearfulness and antidote for vaccination and recurrent colds from over-heating.

September 15th, 1937. Gaining weight—is now 3 st. 7 lbs.—a gain of 11 lbs. in a year. Constipation cured, can eat anything now; gets suddenly tired still, and is dark under the eyes, heavy body odour when asleep; a cervical gland enlarged again during the summer, no sick turns, not so excited—mastoid scar sound.

The child still requires treatment, but her mental symptoms have vastly improved, she is now bearable to live with and not such a strain on her parents and relations; more obedient, not fidgety and not so restless. The fits of anger and rage were only mentioned to me on the second visit, when they had practically ceased.—She gets on well at school now, and has hardly been absent from school since Easter, 1937. *Tuberculinum* Koch 1m, again prescribed.* This child under homœopathic treatment has done remarkably well; gained extraordinarily well; is bright and cheerful and well behaved. A great difference from the puny, difficult, temperamental child of a year ago. No convalescence was needed; she remained in the same surroundings, all the difference that was made, was the regular homœopathic medication.

Tuberculinum is a wonderful medicine in difficult children; but there are other types of children and other remedies which act as well, if they are homœopathically indicated.

Some years ago, a little girl of 3 or 3½ years was brought to me for constipation; she was very plump and fair, and extremely difficult to examine, she shrieked, would not be touched, her eyes turned glassy, she screamed "I won't undress, I won't undress, I'll hit you, I'll tell my daddy." It required a great deal of persuasion and even right to the end she still went on shrieking and protesting at the top of her voice. Even though her temper was

* Weight on 8th December, 1937: 3 st. 10 lb.; another 3 lb. gain.

like the temper of a *Tuberculinum* child, she had not the make-up; for it does not do to prescribe on one symptom only; one has to take many things into consideration. As I said, she was pale and dumpy and round, and nearly as broad as she was long, she felt the heat, she could not take fat and was very affectionate to the people she was fond of. Altogether different from the dainty Dresden china prettiness of *Tuberculinum*. No, *Pulsatilla* was her remedy and *Pulsatilla* continued for a considerable period improved her agitation and her sudden attacks of vile temper which disturbed the neighbours, until now she is a well behaved little madame of seven, who knows how to control herself.

Yes, we always think of *Pulsatilla* as timid and retiring, but once the lid comes off a *Pulsatilla* nature, they can storm and rage with the best of them, and can make the lives of their parents very unpleasant. They are easily frightened, take unaccountable dislikes to people, are fidgety, changeable, and remarkably irritable.

Another little girl dissolved into violent paroxysms of rage and loud uncontrolled weeping, whenever she had an attack of earache, and would not be touched and have her ear looked at. She threatened her mother, that she would take her bag, pack up and leave her, if she let that nasty doctor examine her. She was only three, and yet this wrestle with her temper had gone on for hours, keeping her mother awake and annoying the neighbours in the flats near by. And *Pulsatilla* 1m given hourly at first for the acute earache (of middle-ear disease), and then at lengthening intervals cleared up the ear so that no operation was necessary and with it the piercing shrieks and the vile temper, so that by next morning there was a penitent, well-behaved little girl.

One sees these kicking, screaming, ill-tempered children frequently in the dentist's chair, or even before, while they are waiting to be seen.

Many a child has been cured of its unreasoning fear of dentists by *Tuberculinum* or *Pulsatilla* or occasionally some other remedy, and once it has been treated it bravely faced the ordeal of having the teeth attended to.

Talking of teeth, reminds me of another young girl about fifteen, when I saw her first. Her teeth had turned black as soon as they came through and they were soft and friable, and she suffered a great deal from toothache and spent a lot of time at

the dentist which she dreaded. But this was not all. Her parents
were very worried about her lack of self-control. She could not
be criticized, she was easily irritated about real or imaginary,
trifling things, very touchy, cross and ugly. The world was all
wrong, she took offence where none was meant, and when she
was angry and indignant, she became impulsive and threw things
at anybody, friend or stranger who had caused her irritation. No
amount of reasoning with her did any good, and she seemed to
get worse, the older she got. The mother and father anxiously
wondered what would happen to her, what mad thing she might
do in one of her impulsive rages. I suggested a trial of Homœopathy, and they did not sneer at it, even though the father was a
chemist, and *Staphisagria* 30 altered the make-up and temperament of this unhappy girl very quickly so that two days after the
first dose this budding woman spontaneously confided to her
mother: "The world is so different; everybody is so kind and
nice to me during the last day or two." She did not know she had
the medicine for her uncontrollable rages, but thought she was
having medicine for her toothache! This improvement was not a
flash in the pan, it continued until she became a happy girl, who
could take a joke and laugh at the many minor slights and dis-
comforts of this life. One shudders to think what her impulsive
rages might have led her into. What she was saved from!

One recalls another girl whom one has had under one's care
since infancy. She must be now 12 or 13. She inherited her
mother's Irish temperament, and many difficult scenes one has
had with her. Irascible, easily alarmed, frightened of pain, frightened of seeing blood, would not allow her ears to be touched,
fought and screamed and scratched, even though her ears were
discharging, would not allow me to look at her throat without
scenes. I used to dread the visits I paid her during her various
childish complaints, whooping cough, and measles and scarlet
fever. Each visit was a penalty, it meant tears and fights and
arguments; she got beside herself with rage. I can still see her
with hot scarlet, flushed cheeks, the dark blue eyes with large
black pupils, the thick mops of closely curled fair hair, standing
out from her head like a halo which would not be controlled,
however much it was brushed, defiantly stamping her feet and
trying to run away, "I won't have my ears syringed." It took
three grown-ups to get her ears syringed, when she was almost
totally deaf from a collection of wax; "a little spitfire," quite

beside herself with rage, quite uncontrollable in her tempers. One did not set out to cure her of unnecessary fits of rages, and her alarms about nothing. One set about to cure the child of her constitutional defects which were of a distinctly tubercular nature. She always had night coughs, took colds easily which flew to her chest at once. There were almost invariably râles and moist sounds in her chest; "I am always rattling inside," she quaintly told me once. Her parents were super-careful of her, protecting her against draughts, treating her like a hot-house plant, piled on her woollies; she wore the thickest double-breasted flannels I have ever seen, and yet she was always chesty. I tried to teach them open-air habits, but they all came to nought against the mother's Irish obstinacy. I made the father build an open-air chalet in the garden, where the children were to sleep all through the summer, the first night she and her brother slept out there, the boy fell out of the hammock and laid his scalp open. Naturally the mother blamed me! and they were packed indoors again. When father opened the windows at night, mother shut them again. It was a case of "difficult mother," almost more than "difficult child" in this instance. How often is that not the case? Bring up the parents, and their children will be brought up as they should be. Often I have found that a difficult child became obedient and lamb-like and much more happy, when for some reason or other he or she was separated from the mother. Once an intractable child became positively good-natured and angelic—when her mother died in child-birth, and the girl was taken over and brought up by her aunt. To go back to our Irish colleen; it took years of patience and careful handling of the mother before she could be brought to see—with the tactful help of the father—that fresh air and hardening of the child were most essential in preventing colds, even more so in one who had a tendency to consumption. The cutaneous skin tests that were done confirmed the diagnosis. She had *Tuberculinum* with very little effect; then she got *Drosera* for her night cough which was worse and always disturbed the father in the latter part of the night, and lo and behold, not only did the cough improve and the rattles disappear; but also her tempers improved out of all knowledge. Later on she had *Kali carb.* for right-sided bronchitis with stitching pains which seemed worse in the early morning; and the difficult, very temperamental child became quite calm and philosophical; and when she developed a discharge from her middle ear, and the parents brought her home from boarding school for me to see it, I found she submitted to probing and examining and treating the ear with very good grace, and only a few silent tears rolled down her cheeks. A wonderful alteration in her temperament. And I learned that *Drosera*, a tubercular remedy—is also good for tempestuous children, provided the rest of the symptoms agree. By-the-by, a few doses of *Silica* in a high potency cleared up the discharge and helped to cure the perforated drum in under a month. No local treatment was used, except gently drying out the ear whenever it started to discharge, this ceased entirely after a few days. *Silica* is a remedy closely related to tubercular conditions and septic infections. It is of great use therefore in discharging ears, provided the discharge is not of too offensive a character, when other remedies may be called for. Even septic conditions need to be studied individually so as to find the right remedy corresponding to all the symptoms present.

MORE ABOUT DIFFICULT CHILDREN

THE tubercular constitution seems to produce tempestuous children. *Tuberculinum* loves being out in cold winds, loves battling with storms; the physical likes are closely related to the mental characteristics. Wild tempers, rages and storms internally as well as externally; and they will be wiped out by the correct remedy. Now there is another remedy belonging to the same family, and that is *Phosphorus*: He also is vehement, easily roused to anger, irascible, apprehensive and fearful of many things. I knew a boy who was practically an only child, born after many years, so that there were nearly eighteen years between the two children; naturally he was made much of; and unfortunately he was delicate as a youngster and was spoilt. So he grew up almost unmanageable, was difficult in school; suddenly he would be taken with fits of anger, when nothing could be done with him; would not talk at all; he would rush out of the room, lock himself into a lavatory, often the only place of solitude in a working-class family, and refuse to come out, or even answer his mother when she implored him to be sensible. He would tremble and shake with fear, shout and scream; was frightened of people, scared when alone, frightened of the dark; scared out of his wits during a thunderstorm. Indifferent to the school, indifferent to friends; would only learn when he felt like it; would not go to the doctor or attend at the light clinic for his anæmia. The mother was in despair. She was ordered to take him to a psychological clinic, but she could not get him there; he hid and kicked and shouted when dragged out of his hiding place. In the end he consented to come to me; he was by now a boy of twelve, and had known me since he was an infant, and perhaps I was not so terrifying to him as a complete stranger. Undersized, thin and slim, fair complexioned, red haired, sensitive to noise and touch, very fidgety; could not sit or stand still; felt the cold intensely, liked sympathy and wanted to be made a fuss of. He was so typically *Phosphorous* that I quickly recognized it; and on looking up the records, I found he had

Phosphorus in the past, and on enquiry, his mother related that he always improved rapidly after a week or two of this medicine and would be quite changed and happy, willing to learn, willing to do as he was told, and his nervous fears would disappear completely. For two or three years he came irregularly, whenever he had a turn of the "shakes," and when the school reported he was stubborn and unmanageable.

In time he will grow out of these turns, as long as he gets helped by *Phosphorous* in small doses. I understand he is doing well at school at the moment, and is actually growing big and fat. I wish his mother would bring him regularly and have him definitely attended to monthly. She is a busy working-class woman and until the boy becomes unmanageable, she lets things slide. Such a pity for the boy's sake. His sensitive nature, the sudden unreasonable fears will master him, and he will be a misery to himself and an anxiety to his mother, unless he gets an understanding doctor, armed with the power that Homœopathy gives to her devotees.

Closely related to *Tuberculinum* and *Phosphorus* is *Silica*, though very different in some respects. It has also a difficult nature. I am thinking now of a little boy; he looked a freak and was freakish mentally. Thin, white, almost the colour of chalk, transparent, enormous head, especially the forehead, and the crown drawn out into a peak, a hydrocephaloid head—a child resembling in type to the scrofula of the older physicians, combined with rickets, large, prominent belly, weak legs, especially ankles. I was told he was 18 months or more, before he learned to walk. Constitutionally, he was rickety and feeble as well, timid, retiring, inclined to shirk everything; but when you spoke to him, he became cross and cried, obstinate and headstrong; the more kindly he was spoken to, the more he cried, always hanging on to his mother's skirts. Such a set to, when his throat was about to be examined, not so much kicking and screaming as in a *Tuberculinum* child; more an obstinate, retiring way. "I won't do as you tell me to"—mouth tightly shut, a sullen attitude and then quiet weeping—he would not speak to me for months at his weekly visits. All at once, one day he became bold and to show off and prove his friendliness, he pushed me and slapped my face. He got embarrassed after this episode and refused to speak again for several visits; but he was quietly insistent on being weighed every time he came, and would not go until the sister attended to him—tendency to head sweats and moist feet, offensive foot sweats in the summer and constipation which improved along with the other symptoms. Hated to be touched, had fits of temper, quarrelled with older brother. Multiple perforations of right ear drum, grooved sternum, winged scapula and shoulder blade. Such a worrier, little things troubled him ever so much. Felt the cold very much. *Silica* 30 was given; frequent recurrent colds at first and tonsillitis when first seen on April 11th, 1935; medicine repeated whenever necessary. Bronchitis, September 5th, 1935; sweating head again, lungs full of moist sounds. *Silica* 30 t.d.s. for a week. In December, 1935, developed severe attacks of choking for which he had *Ant. tart.* 30 t.d.s., and *Sulph.* 30 after the bronchitis had disappeared; had a severe choking cough during Christmas, and was feverish for several days; always takes a chill whenever he goes out; had *Arsenic* 30 nightly for this cough. January 23rd, 1936 : very nervous, easily scared. At the beginning for several months he refused to be weighed—weighed 3 st. 3 lbs. 3 ozs. (six years old now). *Tuberculinum* 30 was interposed, as it works well with *Silica.* He had weekly doses of *Tub.* 30; it livened him up; he became more energetic and not so nervous; but his weight remained stationary. Fresh chill started on February 18th. February 25th, measles developed, subsequently seized with paroxysmal choking cough, for which he was given *Drosera* 30, in unit dose. March 5th, getting on; no cough. Measles of course cleared in under the week. March 12th, *Drosera* 30 again; weight 3 st. 3 lbs. 4 ozs.; no loss of weight in spite of measles; gained ½ lb. the next week, and on April 2nd weighed 3st. 4 lbs. 12 oz.—gain of 1½ lbs. in three months. April 23rd, weight 3 st. 5 lbs. 4 ozs. *Drosera* 30 (once) again. May 14th, weight 3 st. 5 lbs. 12 ozs. Nervous of children in playground, head sweats again; *Silica* 30. July 9th, after a month in Clacton, no gain in weight. Shape of head altering; very well and lively. He continued on repeated doses of *Silica* until his weight on September 17th, 1936, was 3 st. 8 lbs. 8 ozs.; he had gained over 5 lbs. in eight months in spite of measles and bronchitis.

Gradually on *Silica* he picked up, and then we found all at once he was growing up, becoming less babyish, would speak up for himself, come along to the dispensary without his mother, talk and chatter with the other children and now, when he is eight, his body is well covered, he has put on well over 8 lbs. this last year; he is not catching colds as frequently as he used to; he does not look so transparent, and is becoming an independent little man; his head is still peaked and on the large size; he is still pallid and fair skinned, but the whole family is like that.

If he had not had Homœopathy, he would have grown up into a shrinking, timid man, that is, if he did not die from his bronchitis first!—with no spunk, no self-confidence, lack of grit, weak and embarrassed, dreading to do anything on his own responsibility. What a wonderful thing *Silica* is in building up the body as well as the mind!

Now we shall leave the tubercular family and go to another group. The *Baryta carb.* child is very similar, both in appearance and in temperament to the *Silica* nature. It has a big head, big abdomen, thin legs, and tendency to enlarged glands and enlarged tonsils, not septic or suppurating tonsils but more general inflammation and enlargement with each cold. A painfully shy child, sits about in corners, hides behind his mother; even as a baby he hides his face in his hands, as if he was afraid or ashamed. Cowardly, irresolute, bashful, afraid of strangers, does not want to play with other children, sits in a corner by himself, constantly whining. We had such a boy, dwarfish in mind as well as in body; would not answer or speak when spoken to; he was eight when I first met him, he could not read or would not read, I was never sure which it was, looked at me with his brown eyes and perhaps five minutes later, if at all, he would stammeringly bring a word out. For weeks it was like that; he was always stammering, if he answered at all. At school they could do nothing with him; he was much too frightened and shy; bullied by his older sister, he was a poor, mentally unstable person who could never string even a short sentence together without a stammer. What an existence and prospect for that lad! *Baryta carb.* did a great deal for him; and during the eighteen months he attended regularly, he gained well in stature and weight, and actually gave up stammering and showed that he could read; he talked quite freely with his schoolmates, and was even seen fighting with another boy in the street. Alas, the slum-clearing scheme removed him from that area, and I lost sight of him. I am very much afraid his improvement will not be maintained without the stimulating and vitalizing effect of the *Baryta carb.*

I remember a fellow-woman student who was afflicted with

this most painful silence and shyness. She was a few years older and further on than myself, so I came very little in contact with her, but I never saw her speak to anybody; and if any professor or doctor looked at her even, she would blush and look away and never answer. She was a standing joke at college, and how she ever plucked up enough courage to answer the examiners, I do not know; the legend went that she never said one word to any of the students she was with for the whole five years of her course. And however she managed to get on as a medical woman in practice, I cannot imagine!

Then there was that little boy of four, whose medical story I have told already in these pages, who had been treated for six months at the clinic of a well-known children's specialist with gallipots of cod liver oil and malt, without any appreciable effect on his nerves, his weight or his unresolved pneumonia following on scarlet fever and diphtheria. He weighed 26 lbs. in October, 1933; in August, 1934, his weight was 35 lbs. and from being a shy, nervous boy, who would not look at a stranger, would not play with other children, hiding himself in a corner, never a word out of him, he developed into a bright, cheerful, playful soul, full of fun and gaiety. First a few doses of *Kali carbonicum* were given for his unresolved right-sided basal pneumonia, and then *Baryta carb.* 6 night and morning for some weeks, followed by *Baryta carb m.* They suggested psychological treatment for him and an observation centre for his peculiar ways; Homœopathy so vitalized him and changed him, that he gained 9 lbs. in ten months, lost his cough and his pneumonic patch, and his terrible shyness and fear of strangers. Is it not worth while to be a homœopath psychologist? I still see his mother sometimes; they have moved out of the district, and he is getting on very well in school, a bright, active child, up to all the usual boyish tricks!

I personally have never seen such results in such a short time, as a student or as a house surgeon in the out-patients' departments of children's hospitals, with the usual tonics such as Parrish's food, strychnine and quinine mixtures, oil and malt, and the other unpalatable concoctions. If I had, I should certainly never have troubled to learn and study Homœopathy; it means much burning of midnight oil, concentrated hard work. But the results are worth it. I only wish that Homœopathy were better known, and that more doctors would get over their prejudice and investigate it.

Now for another shy, difficult child, and quite different from the *Baryta carb.* nature. This is *Natrum muriaticum*, or common salt. Common salt is in such general use in everyday life that many people, especially doctors, cannot and will not believe that it can be of any use in the minute doses we give it in. Dr. Burnett was very keen on it and went fully into the uses of *Natrum mur.* and wrote a book on the dynamic uses of *Nat. mur.*, as we call it, lovingly and shortly. The *Nat. mur.* child is late learning to walk, late in learning to talk; sometimes a boy is four years and older, before he even opens his lips to speak. As far as I know, whenever an anxious mother takes such a dumb child to the children's specialist, she is always told that there is nothing to worry about, he will grow out of it. He will do so in most cases, but very slowly; but give him *Nat. mur.*, or it might be some other remedy, just as the combination of symptoms demand it, and the child will suddenly find his tongue and begin to chatter as if to the manner born. *Natrum mur.* is usually a pale child with a greasy, waxy, shiny skin; emaciated, weak, thin, eats well and yet does not put on any weight. I knew such a boy; one of several, he wanted to be left alone; if anybody talked to him, he would turn his face to the wall; he would weep and shed bitter tears when reprimanded or looked at; the more he was sympathized with, the more he cried; he used to cry with annoyance, sympathy made him worse, hated being fussed over, he used to get so angry and bellow and shriek with anger. Backward in learning; slow, a fearful dunce, awkward and clumsy, always letting things drop, always stumbling when walking; he was nearly two before he learnt to walk and nearly four before he deigned to speak; frightened of burglars, startled at noise, on suddenly hearing a door open. Craving for salt, but did not like fat; scared of thunder; his lips easily cracked and split, especially in the middle of the lower lip, and when he was nine years old he developed a terrible divergent strabismus (squint), for which the surgeons wished to operate. He feels the cold, and he is never at his best in the mornings; does not wake until the day has got warmed up a bit, that is until after 10 a.m. What a dunce he was in school! *Nat. mur.* did wonders for him. His awkwardness, mental as well as physical, left him; he became much brighter in school, suddenly made great strides in his lessons and even his squint improved. One wonders, if he can only be kept away from the surgeons for another six months, whether his eyes might not become straight again. Why not? More wonderful things have happened. Squint, after all, is unequal pulling and straining of the muscles in different directions, due to weakness; and when nature is stimulated by the correctly indicated remedy, the *vis medicatrix naturæ* will do the rest. I have seen several boys, emaciated, thin, dunces at school, almost mentally deficient, make tremendous strides under *Natrum muriaticum*, the dynamized common salt. Unfortunately it means hunting through hundreds of records sometimes, and one does not remember the names; only the broad medical facts and the faces. Perhaps, if I get some leisure, I shall find some more of these salt cases, which are rather intriguing. When you consider that salt in physiological doses makes no change in the child, but give it in a high potency —it does not work below the 6th centesimal dilution, and does better in the 30th, I think—it begins to change them mentally and physically. But again remember : the salt characteristics must be present. You must individualize; consider each child, each person who comes to you. Children are very inarticulate, but sometimes you do get an intelligent mother who can tell you the idiosyncrasies of her child, who has watched over it lovingly and with care; and then you do get wonderful results, much more striking than with adults, whose symptoms have so often been suppressed and muddled up and mixed up with so many other things. You do not often get such a stupid mother as the following, who told me she gave her boy every night on going to bed a dose of some kind of aspirin preparation in hot milk, so as to make him sleep. "Aspirin," I exclaimed in great horror, "but that is a very strong medicine to give, it weakens the heart eventually, it depresses the nervous system, it suppresses all the symptoms and by oxydizing the oxygen in the cells, it kills the individual cells and devitalizes the body." She would not believe me, of course, when I told her all this. The posters everywhere screamed of the benefits that particular patent remedy gave to those who patronized it, that she was ruining the child's nervous system and undermining its health, was nothing to her. "It was only a fad of mine. She had seen it with her own eyes, in black and white, what this drug could do, and nothing I said convinced her I was right," she said. Of course, I told her straight, I could do her child no good, and I refused to treat him, as long as she carried on with this medicine. She went on her way unrepenting and scorned my advice. Poor deluded woman, poor child to have such a blind mother. I object to all the different pain killers which are so frequently the cause of accidental suicides who unwittingly take an overdose. These should all be cast out far into the ocean, where they will only kill the fish, instead of killing and underminig the health and the will power of so many useful lives. The indicated homœpathic remedy will do better work than all the sleeping-draughts and anodynes.

Let us hie back to our difficult children. In October, 1935, a boy of nine was brought to me with the following symptoms: he was a great trial and anxiety to his parents, cruel and spiteful and jealous and suspicious to a degree, pinched and tormented cats and dogs, pinched and hurt and nearly killed his young sister by squeezing her, because he was jealous of her; a wanderer, tried to run away from home once or twice; bit his nails; had occasional nocturnal enuresis (bed-wetting); defaecated into his knickers until quite recently, until he was told he would not get a Sunday suit, but would have to wear his dirty trousers, until he improved. As he was rather vain, he quickly decided to be good; it was all naughtiness, he was not mentally deficient. Had fits of temper, shouted and screamed, bit, called people all sorts of names; insolent and rude when spoken to, very silly and giggly, and laughed inordinately at times about nothing; fits of being very affectionate and then kissed everybody; liked new things, made himself very busy and liked to show off, not shy with strangers, but quiet and well behaved—extremely so when he came in to me. There was only a suspicious sideways glance at me, when I talked to him; wanted to know why I wanted him to undress, but decided he did not wish to be examined. Stole everything he could lay hands on in school; went into the larder and helped himself to food, very fond of sugar and sweets and jams. Had an accident and crushed his fingers in the door of a motor-car four years ago; scared and frightened of cars ever since. Fear of being alone, fear of a mirror, fear of going near water; fear of thunderstorms. *Stramonium* has all these symptoms and *Stramonium* 30 was given. I forgot to mention, he got on very badly at school, was no good at arithmetic; had periods "of being blank" at school, and I think he had been turned out of two or three different schools as being too peculiar and difficult. Felt the cold, had perspiring hands and feet. Seen again at the end of November, irresponsible, spiteful, smacks the face of his sister, impulsive, drags and pulls her hair out; has screaming fits when he does not get the things he wants; rude and rough at school, kicks other children; sudden storms of rage. *Stramonium* 30 repeated.

December 1935. Hates contradiction, screams when thwarted, no sense of right or wrong, spiteful. *Stramonium* 30 night and morning. January 8th, 1936: found out that there was tuberculosis in the family; also tonsils and adenoids. Much steadier, brighter, not so scared or suspicious. I was able to examine him for the first time. Some improvement at last! *Tuberculinum* 30 in occasional doses and *Stramonium* 30 every morning. January 27th, 1936: Great improvement, much brighter, answers very intelligently. *Tuberculinum* 30 again, and Stramonium 30 every morning on rising. March 3rd, 1936: Very tired afternoons; always laughing, cannot stop laughing, shouts like mad if contradicted; afraid of feathers and of spiders; has no ideas of numbers. Microcephalic. *Stramonium* 48m. weekly. April 25th, 1936: Getting on well at school; still very jealous of sister, and excitable; afraid of thunderstorms. Repeat *Stramonium* 48m. weekly. June 17th, 1936: Much improved all round. *Stramonium* 48m. bi-weekly for a month. July 17th, 1936: Great improvement; very sulky still; hates his sisters and mother. *Fluoric acid* 30.

I have not seen the boy since, but have heard from an outsider that he is doing well and getting on very nicely at school.

A *Stramonium* child with all the *Stramonium* peculiarities, but the indicated remedy, *Stramonium*, did not get to work until the underlying constitution—tuberculosis—was tackled; then we got him on very rapidly. Then later on, the deep lying family hatred was revealed, and *Fluoric acid* was prescribed; did it finish the case and cure it entirely? People have an aggravating habit of not letting you know, and you are left wondering. The child was to have been sent down from school, as being too impossible; after the *Stramonium*, the school reports were good, and he was kept on. I surmise the improvement continued.

A friend of mine reproved me very much for not having mentioned the *"Chamomilla"* child among the "difficult children". She looked for *Chamomilla* straight away and was very puzzled at not finding any reference made to it.

Now I had a very good reason for omitting *Chamomilla* so far, and mentioning the *Chamomilla* child as a difficult child. To make myself clear I want to explain in detail the make-up of

Chamomilla. It has an ugly, cussed temperament; it is nervy, is easily angered and capricious, can't be spoken to, *won't* be touched, is obstinate, self-willed, easily chagrined. But the great characteristic is that there is a definite physical reason for all this cussed, ugly behaviour, for this chagrin, for the anger and the irritability. It is an acute remedy and you only get the *Chamomilla* symptoms if *there is* PAIN *present.* You get all these peculiarities in the teething children, either in infancy or later on during the second dentition, with the colic during teething, with earache, neuralgia, headaches, in menstrual pain, and the labour pains of the lying-in woman. The great outstanding feature is hypersensitiveness to pain, oversensitive, snappy with pain, suffers intensely from the slightest ache. They will call out "This pain is more than I can bear, can't something be done?" You find a *Chamomilla* child with the pangs of an erupting tooth asking daddy to carry him, then he holds out his arms to mammy, then he goes to nanny or back to daddy. He calls out for his teddy bear, if he can speak, and when he gets it, he throws it in one corner, "Don't want it; want my motor engine." He throws that down when it is given to him, wants his dinner and then throws his plate across the table. Nothing pleases him, nothing is right; shrieks and howls if he is not carried. His cheeks are red, sometimes only one side of his face is red; his face is hot, while the rest of the body is cold. Sweating of the head and scalp. The pains and tempers are always worse after 9 o'clock at night, from 9 o'clock until midnight, and sometimes 9 o'clock in the morning. He is not one to suffer any pain in silence. Everybody else must suffer with him, his shrieks at night are so penetrating that he exhausts the patience of his father. In the working-class quarters, the friends and neighbours are so sure that the poor child is being maltreated that frequently the "Cruelty-to-Children" officer is called in and the poor, innocent parents have to put up with the ignominy of being visited by the "Cruelty man" to account for the shrieking child. Thus insult is added to injury! No wonder that the distracted mother rushes to the out-patients' department of the nearest hospital in order to beg for a soothing draught! She usually gets Chloral, which has the desired effect, it acts on the brain-cells and is a powerful dope. Naturally Homœopaths do not approve of this drug as it anæsthetizes and temporarily anyway paralyses the nerve cells of the brain and spinal cord. How much simpler are our remedies, they are innocuous and do act just as well, if not better, without poisoning and damaging the all-important nuclei of the grey matter of the brain. One wishes that the medical profession would deign to study our pharmacopœia and try out our remedies.

It is curious how different people react to pain. One sees this well marked in the way people behave during labour. I remember the stoic woman, who quietly walked up and down the room, biting her lips and there was never a murmur, never a sigh even until the very end, when just a slight groan escaped her, for which she apologized. And she was only a poor coster woman! I admired her self-control. And on the other hand there is the *Chamomilla* woman; over-sensitive to pain, and she lets you know it, too! She screams, she shouts, she throws herself about, she hits you, punches you, pulls your hair, until the poor doctor or nurse is black and blue all over. She is in such agonies of pain that she really does not know what she is doing. But give her some *Chamomilla*, and you alter her at once. She becomes docile and quiet and the labour pains seem to become much easier and the mental unrest and irritability are gone. *Chamomilla* anger and irascibility always reminds me of a sudden April shower and April storm, it is short and sharp while it lasts, and aggravating, but it is over soon and the sun shines in between. The baby and the toddler with his toothache and his colic will forget all about his pain and his anger, as soon as it is over, and will be all smiles, and will be amiable, especially if he gets some *Chamomilla*. In coffee-drinking countries, as in the United States, in Germany, in France, one often comes across *Chamomilla* symptoms and *Chamomilla* patients. Coffee and *Chamomilla* are antidotes—one to the other.

Let me repeat it, *Chamomilla* symptoms are associated with pains and a child that requires *Chamomilla* is not a real "difficult child". When the cause is removed, when the tooth is through, the pain ceases, the irritability goes, and the storm is over.

Another criticism reached me, this time from America, suggesting that difficult children were called "Problem children" there. I stand corrected, for the psychologists do call them problem children, for many do present rather serious problems to the psychologist, and it means long periods of observation and close study of the behaviour of each child before a course of treatment can be suggested by the psychologist. The general physician, unless he is trained in psychological methods, can do very little except shrug his shoulders and suggest that the child will probably grow out of it. Now I claim that the Homœopaths are better psychologists than the psychologists themselves, at any rate they were taught to consider each individual as a unit, to be separately watched, observed and studied long before the rest of the profession thought fit to do so. And they also possess positive means of curing psychological problems: i.e. by way of the indicated remedy. Hahnemann, our founder, taught his disciples to pay attention to the mental, as he calls it, symptoms—which correspond to the modern time psychological re-actions. Thus we have collected pages and pages of psychological symptoms, produced by the healthy prover of a remedy and following on the principles of the law "that like cures like"—the same symptoms found in the sick, that is mentally or psychologically infirm or abnormal persons will be cured by the similar remedy. Hence a difficult child does not present such a "problem" to the true follower of Hahnemann as to the psychologist.

Let me present a few such problem children, if you like to call them so. Some children are made difficult by their surroundings, by the wrong methods of training, or lack of training and discipline; but others are "erblich belasted"—as the Germans term it —have a hereditary weakness passed on through either mother or father. I remember a very sad case which I heard, when I was a child myself—a child with rather long ears I am afraid— who heard more than she was meant to, I am sure. The young mother came from a very good family and married beneath her against her family's wishes. The result was, she was cast off, and unfortunately the young husband immediately lost his job and the couple very often suffered from hunger and went through very hard days, suffered so badly that she often stood outside the baker's and the hotels, wishing she could go in and steal the food to appease her hunger. When the little boy was born, and grew up to about four or five years of age, he started to thieve and nothing would make any difference. No punishments, no gentle reprimands; he belonged to the light-fingered brigade. And the older he grew the worse his thieving propensities became. The mother had become reconciled to her parents and the other children were quite normal except the unfortunate firstborn. Nothing could be done with him, and he was taken before the magistrate who sent him to the penitentiary for corrective training. I do not recall whether by strict discipline at the Industrial School this unfortunate psychological misfit outgrew his inherited tendencies, but he could have been cured by homœopathic treatment. We have fifteen remedies to choose from for Kleptomania. I have not come in personal contact since with cases of irresistible tendency to stealing; but if I should, I should know how to approach the subject.

There are other psychological misfits I have met with, since I have passed the apprentice stage in Homœopathy.

A little girl was first seen at two years and six months. She only weighed 23 lbs., was about 7 lbs. underweight, and had spent nearly eighteen months in a large children's hospital, where she had treatment for rickets. She was still wearing surgical boots for greenstick fractures of her leg bones. She was a dirty child, totally untrained and dirty in her habits, with attacks of wicked temper and mentally backward, could not understand what was being said to her. She was put on cod liver oil, 1 dessert-spoonful twice daily, which the foster-mother religiously carried out. The child was one of the unwanted "strays" of this world. The mother had been infected with venereal disease and the infant was born in a Lock hospital. The foster-mother, one of the practical saints of this world, a great child lover who had a nursery full of unwanted children, whom she gets through various rescue societies, and whom she strives unceasingly to make into healthy boys and girls. Alas, with but indifferent success! At three years eight months this little misery weighed only 27 lbs. 12 ozs., she had a tremendous appetite, was always eating enormous meals, and still remained 7 lbs. underweight for her age. On these symptoms she was given *Sulphur* 30 for a time, but three months later the weight was still the same, even though she had plenty of milk, plenty of good food, and three teaspoons of cod liver oil daily. The foster-mother reported three months later, when she was four years old, that the child was very secretive and destructive, scratched windows with flints, lied and stole things out of drawers, and hid the articles, and then denied having done so. I did not see her again until the beginning of October 1937 when the foster-mother reported that she was still stealing and was always setting things on fire. I remembered the family history of syphilitic infection and asked her to be brought along for an examination. She was over five years old and weighed 33 lbs.

7 ozs., still 9 lbs. underweight, looked pale and undersized, a great eater—psychological report, bites other children, throws things out of the windows, is quarrelsome, lies and steals things from the school and is always setting things on fire in the house. The syphilitic family history and the tendency of setting things on fire, and the bold, naughty behaviour, quarrelsome, etc., gave me the remedy : *Hepar sulph.*, which she was given. No other alterations were made in diet or mental treatment. She was seen again on January 6th, 1938, when she was found to have gained 2¼ lbs., in three months ! She had taken eight months previously to put on 2¼ lbs.; there was a distinct improvement in the general metabolism; the child looked well, had a good colour and was much brighter. She had made no further attempt to light matches or set the house on fire. The foster-mother could not make it out and she thought she had been more carefully supervised ! She had several doses of *Hepar sulph.* in a high potency. She still requires further treatment; but the unpleasant tendency of fire raising has been controlled; and the rest, the love for stealing sweets and dainties, will be controlled in a short time. It is very interesting to find how quickly Homœopathy acts, *if one gets the right remedy.* This child, of course, with a syphilitic mother, a father who is rarely sober, is much to be pitied, and is very poor stuff to try and improve and build on. One has need of psychological treatment for these fire raisers, but I do not remember how long a time is required before a cure is achieved. My experience is, that these psychological cases take years before any appreciable improvement takes place. I may be wrong; but I think Homœopathy compares very favourably as regards the time taken to bring about a cure.

HOMŒOPATHY IN WOMEN'S AILMENTS

THE number of unnecessary operations performed on hapless women in the course of a year all over England must go into many, many thousands. I came across a poor woman today, white, bloodless, haggard, who told me a pitiful tale. Never well since the birth of her child eighteen months ago, frequent attacks of hæmorrhage, several periods of many weeks spent in hospital. Her inside had been "cleaned out", as she called it, several times. Now she was sent home to recuperate for the next big operation : removal of some more of her organs. She took it as a matter of course, was rather proud of it than otherwise, and her case is one of many.

I learned long ago that Homœpathy can do a great deal for these poor sufferers, even in apparently hopeless cases. Many years ago, in my early youth, when I was waiting for work to drop in, a woman was brought in by her friends. She was almost in a state of collapse, thin, elderly, sallow, with deep lines of suffering and pain on her face, a typical uterine complexion. I said to myself : "What could I do for her ?" I asked her what she complained of : Oh, she had a terrible big lump in her groin which made it difficult for her to walk or sit down. On examination, I found a mass bigger than a cricket ball in the fork of her legs, a complete prolapse of the female organs. She had been many times to the big general hospital nearby and was the despair of the dressers and of the young doctors. The pessary, the uterine support, put in during the morning, would be out before eventide many times. She had been given the largest supports they had in stock, and not one would "stay put". She had been ordered to have an operation to stitch up the prolapsed organs, but had flatly refused. Now she came to me to get some help.

I was in a predicament. My medical training said : "Operation is the only thing." My knowledge of homœopathic drugs whispered : "Try the indicated remedy." The organ was replaced, and the pessary put in, and with fear and trembling a dose of *Sepia* 1,000 potency was given on her history and such few symptoms as I could get out of the poor, distracted, pain-racked woman; mainly on her physical appearance, yellow liver spots on her face, great depression, irritability, a great sufferer from the cold.

I expected to have her back on my doorstep very soon. Nothing happened. Day after day went by, and she did not appear. She had gone to hospital, and had her operation after all, I thought. Three months later a bright, pink and white complexioned woman, middle-aged, came in, and introduced two new patients to me. "Don't you remember me?" It was my wreck of a woman with a prolapse. "Have you had your operation?" "Oh, no!" was the reply. "I have still got the ring in. I feel so different, so happy and full of energy." I could hardly believe my eyes. The incredible had been achieved. The ligaments and muscles of the pelvic floor had tightened up and had kept the pessary in. She wore the pessary for six months or so, and after this we dispensed with it entirely. The prolapse never came back as long as I knew her. This was for about seven years. This woman had been saved from a dangerous operation and from a tedious and long-drawn-out convalescence at the cost of what? A single powder of *Sepia* 1,000 potency which only required to be repeated at six months intervals.

After this case my work consisted largely in saving people from unnecessary surgical operations. There was a dark-haired young girl of 19 or 20, full-blooded, with scanty menstrual flow, intense dragging-down pains in her abdomen. She had a displaced uterus, suffered from severe pains in the forehead with disturbance of vision, pain in the bottom of the back, the sacrum; great suffering during menstrual periods, great heats in the head, emptiness of stomach and hot soles of feet. All her symptoms were very like *Sulphur*. Yet she was irritable with it, could not speak a decent word to anybody even in the office, could not bear sympathy, and withal was like a *Pulsatilla* patient, for she could not stand a warm room and liked to be out in the cold. This patient had been told by a surgeon that she required a curetting for intense suffering at the menstrual periods and probably later an operation to fix the misplaced uterus. One or two doses of *Lilium tigrinum* in a high potency relieved her suffering, so that she could attend to her work and laugh at the thoughts of an operation. This is the way to individualize remedies, compare and contrast.

And what about the dozens of young girls with acute menstrual pains, with sickness and vomiting and scanty periods, with times of silent agony, bitter wrangling with fate for having put all this suffering, month after month, on one to bear! What is the usual advice given to such an unfortunate being? Again an operation which may help her for five or six months, and then a return of the agony. In many cases all that is wanted is a dose or two of *Pulsatilla*, or *Sulphur*, or *Sepia*—if only the poor victims knew—without any degrading examination even.

Readers should not think that the cures described offer any exceptional features, or that they require any exceptional ability on the part of the prescriber. Mr. Ellis Barker has collected in his book, *Miracles of Healing,* hundreds of similar cures of gynecological and other diseases, performed by more than a hundred homœopathic doctors. They are everyday events in the lives of homœopaths, and I am sure, there are dozens of homœopaths who could have done just as well as I have done. Furthermore, it is not necessary to treat such cases with single, or very rare, doses of medicine in a high potency. A number of doses in a low or medium potency would have done just as well.

Surgery should be the handmaiden of Medicine. In the olden days right up to the eighties, the physician was more highly respected than his brother the surgeon; indeed, the pompous physician, complete with snuff-box, which he used to keep off bad humours and fevers—wig and golden-headed cane, looked down on the barber surgeon whom he only employed in a menial position, i.e. in the frequent blood-lettings fashionable at the time, and perhaps for the crushing operations for stone in the bladder. Otherwise surgery was very little known, except for amputations for gunshot wounds and fractures on the battlefields. Most of these operations were unsuccessful, as the patients succumbed in large numbers to wound fevers due, as we know now, to sepsis.

No wonder that a surgeon was only called in as a very last resort. All this changed completely after the discoveries of such brilliant men as Semmelweiss of Vienna who found the cause of puerperal fevers which ravaged the maternity hospitals in those days—of Pasteur, who first discovered bacteria—of Lister, who made surgical operations no longer playthings of chance by using antiseptics to kill the fatal bacteria—of Simpson, who first used

anæsthetics, and thus took away the ghastly horror of consciousness of pain. The combined effects of these discoveries helped
surgery on enormously. The surgeon became bolder, as patients
survived their manipulations, and more and more brilliant operations were invented, as the technique improved, and nowadays
surgery has reached its zenith.

Operations on the heart, the lungs, the spleen and the brain
are daily performed successfully, as far as the surgeon is concerned. It has become a mechanical job, one wonders if the
patient is not often a minor consideration, and his pains, his dis-
abilities are as great, if not worse, after the operation than they
were previously. Certain indefinite symptoms are present in the
patient; he has caught a germ, it is said; his appendix, he is told,
must be removed. It is done; months go by; still the same unpleasant symptoms recur; now the blame is put on the gall-
bladder—or it may be *vice versa*—and is brilliantly dealt with.
Still the patient feels ill or is never well; some other part of his
anatomy is investigated and fixed upon as being useless, may indeed be fatal to him, he is told if left; it might be his tonsils or
his frontal sinus or even a large part of his bowels may have to
be sacrificed at the altar of the great god Moloch, and so the
merry race goes on. Alas! that surgery only is considered for so
many ailments, for only the products of the disease are removed
by the knife, the actual cause of all the trouble is not touched
and is still the same as it was before the operation and continues
to act. It is no wonder, that most young medical men go in for
surgery; the kudos are much greater and something definite is
being done: while until recently there was very little treatment
for a medical case except, "refer to a surgeon".

A well-known brilliant surgeon in Dublin who excelled in most
out-of-the-way, venturesome operations, spoke very slightingly to
me years ago of the uselessness of medicines. "They are all rubbish and should be thrown overboard, with the exception of perhaps one or two pain-killing drugs. You don't believe in medicines, do you?" he turned to me, then the young tyro just fresh
from the schools. I suppose he saw the faintly doubting expres-
sion in my face. "Oh, no," I quickly replied, with a proviso in
my mind—it would not do to offend the great man. Certainly I
did not believe in the efficacy of the medicines, as I had seen
them applied in the wards of the famous hospital, where I was

trained. They might just as well not have been given. The expectant treatment, the do-nothing and leave-it-to-nature method, did just as well and very often better than drastic over-dosing.

Surgery is glamorous, but medicine is more wonderful still if you know how to prevent illness, and how to prevent operations.

Many operations are unnecessary, and even such things as new growths and tumours can be removed without the aid of the knife. This is not an exaggeration or an idle statement.

Tumours have been cured in the past, our homœopathic literature is full of examples, and they are daily being cured now, and more would be cured, if Homœopathy were given a chance. But the surgical technique has developed to such a fine art that only surgery is considered for any case of growth or tumour.

"You must have an operation," the patient is told. "Nonsense, it can't be removed by medicines," if he or she feebly and hesitantly objects, and so they are swept off their feet and into a hospital ward before they have time to look round. Surgeons forget that you may remove the tumour safely, but you do not remove or cure the cause, the original cause in the first instance that produced the tumour. And that can only be done by treating each patient individually, taking the full history in the minutest details, and by building up and rectifying the constitution, the patient is made well and strong, the tendency to grow tumours is put right and frequently, in the majority of the cases, the tumour itself disappears, never to return. In a few cases the tumour may have to be removed surgically, but the patient by that time is fully well and strong, as his health has been built up, and he can stand the operation better.

Years ago I came across such a woman, a patient of the late Dr. Ridpath, who was a very keen Homœopath. She had been treated by him for a large fibroid of the uterus, and she was quite unlike any other fibroid patient I had ever met before. She looked so healthy, so bright and well, she had hæmorrhages, she had palpitations, but all these had stopped : there were no constitutional symptoms, only the foreign body, the large fibroid, was left. She stayed in hospital for three weeks and never turned a hair, and I have never seen a patient get over an operation so easily and quickly. Dr. Ridpath must have been a wonderful Homœopath to implant such faith in his patients and build up their health, so that they could go through operations so well. I rather smiled a smile of disbelief when this lady told me about other cases of fibroids being cured without operations; but youth is rash and condemns quickly.

With greater experience I have come to the conclusion that it is not only probable, but almost certain that fibroids and other tumours can be cured medicinally; but it requires time and patience, and the patient must be willing to keep under treatment and carry out instructions faithfully. The late Dr. Burnett had many brilliant cures of tumours of breast, uterus and other parts of the body to his credit, and his writings are very illuminating. He mentions one cure of a very large fibroid which took three years in the curing and complete removal—by medicines; probably it might have been quicker if the lady had not been so devoted to travelling and had not absented herself sometimes for months. Another case took well over two years; certainly an operation would have been quicker, but people forget the invalidism that follows after an operation, and many people are never the same afterwards. "Is it not much better to leave a patient whole instead of removing a woman's organs wholesale, and leaving her crippled and weakly?"

Listen to this case history:

Mrs. B., aged 41 years, seen first at the end of October 1935. Complains of profuse hæmorrhages. Her medical practitioner discovered uterine fibroids and advised operation. She came for medical treatment instead, having heard what Homœopathy could do. Pale, exsanguinated woman, thin, tired, red lips, round-shouldered and bent. M.P.— $\frac{6}{26}$ + + flow, bright red colour, with dark red clots. Has prolapse of the abdomen for which she has worn a belt for years. Very sensitive to diapers which irritate the skin very much. Short of breath, worse exertion, worse ascending stairs, does not eat fat meat, feels worse about 11 a.m., felt worse during heat of summer; pain in back, mid-scapular region, better resting, better lying down; indigestion, flatulence, swollen and distended feeling after eating, better eructation, has to take bicarbonate of soda for it; very constipated; takes Normacol; on examination found several small fibroids; uterus itself was very heavy, ante-flexed and fibrotic, extended to quite three fingers' breadths above symphysis pubis. Prescribed *Sulphur* 6 t.d.s. on general symptoms.

January 7th, 1936 (two months later). M.P. four days only, clots much less; indigestion much better, not so swollen after food; uterus smaller, only just above symphysis pubis and nodules not so distinct. Heard for the first time that there was a tendency to tuberculosis; had been in a sanatorium for apical tuberculosis; cannot take cod liver oil.

(1) *Tuberculinum* 30. Four powders at weekly intervals.

(2) *Fraxinus americana* Ø. Five drops night and morning.

Fraxinus is one of Dr. Burnett's organ remedies, which he took over from Rademacher, and with which he cured many cases of uterine fibroids and heavy sub-involuted uteri.

Lost sight of patient for six months.

Seen again on July 11th, 1936.

Periods less; feels better during periods; has had no treatment since end of March; constipation improved, does not take Normacol any more; nocturnal frequency has stopped; sputum examined in May; no tuberculosis found. Had influenza in April and cough for weeks afterwards.

M.P. regular $\dfrac{4 \text{ days}}{26 \text{ days}}$ Per. vag.; uterus smaller.

The general practitioner who first discovered the fibroids examined her in April and found to his surprise that the fibroids had practically disappeared. Indigestion much improved, can eat anything now and does not take bicarbonate of soda, as there is no longer any fullness after meals; enjoys going out to dinner now.

Continued *Fraxinus americana* Ø mins.V night and morning.

December 11th, 1936. Much better; uterus small, fibroids appear to have gone. No frequency of micturition, no indigestion; but sick headaches before periods; feels cold now; worse sympathy; better company; fear of being alone in the house; fear of thunderstorms; worse mornings. On the general symptoms she received *Nat. mur.* 30 for her sick headaches, which is an old symptom recurring.

She is still not out of the wood, her constitution has not been completely built up yet, but her fibroids have disappeared.

Unfortunately she is a busy woman and has no time to give to her ailments. If she had been attending more regularly, more likely her constitutional symptoms would have improved more quickly. It is a triumph for Homœopathy to cure fibroids within fourteen months, and at the same time to improve a woman's health so that she can enjoy life more than she ever did before. She is very pleased that she escaped the operation, I am told.

She has been seen again quite recently, and the cure still holds good.

TROUBLES OF THE CHANGE OF LIFE

A GREAT deal of rubbish is written and talked about "The Change".

"A woman is finished after 40," one doctor told a woman patient of mine. I could not quite get his meaning. Did he mean a woman could not bear any more children after 40 and was therefore a useless burden to the man, or did he imply that women automatically became invalids during the menopause and were, therefore, finished and hence no more good to humanity? In neither of these points was that doctor man correct, for I have known women having children long after they were 40.

One woman I remember got married at 39 and had three children during the three following years. Another woman after a twenty-five years' pause came for so-called "disturbances due to change", and I discovered a five months' pregnancy, and she was 53 and a grandmother of several years' standing! We nearly came to blows over it; quite a serious matter for me, as she was a hefty coster-woman and used to fighting with her fists. I calmed the good lady by offering her a good bet on my being right, and her sporting instincts conquered, much to my relief. We became very good friends in the end, and the lusty boy she presented her husband with in due course was much admired in the family. I never got my 5s. though, but saved my reputation, which was of greater value to me.

And what about the number of women who do much valuable work after middle-age as magistrates, J.P.s, on Social Councils and other committees too numerous to mention here? Would you call their work useless? It is quite true that women suffer, and many suffer a great deal during this period of change, and much irreparable damage is done to their constitution by over-drugging and wrong drugging, and years of misery might be saved them if they knew what to do. Beware of patent remedies, away with all the numerous sleeping draughts. Avoid alcohol in any shape or form during these fateful years; a peculiar feeling of exhaustion comes over a woman frequently, and in desperation she takes "a drop" to strengthen herself and to overcome this weakness. "Ah, that touches the spot. I feel so muzzy and this just does it," a Lancashire woman used to say to me. A most dangerous habit this; one drop leads to a glass, and soon a glass leads to a bottle, and the dangerous habit of tippling commences. These cases of drunkenness in women are caused more by this "just taking a drop" than anything else.

But what to do with this feeling of tiredness, this exhaustion, the terrible heats and the flushes, the bursting headaches which all but too commonly accompany the change?

Here Homœopathy is again an invaluable ally. It cures easily and quickly without exposing a woman to any dangers, such as the drugs, belonging to the barbiturates do. There are many of them, which may at first give much relief, but soon the organism gets used to their action. One has to take larger and larger doses, and an over-dose is so easily taken and then—a coroner's inquest.

Remember our homœopathic Materia Medica is full of remedies that fit the menopause.

There is *Sulphur*, that famous polychrest *Sulphur*. We have such symptoms as "Heat on top of the head, flushes in the face, the patient from congestion in the head feels oppressed, she wants windows and doors open, she feels so weak at 11 a.m., a faintness or gone sensation in stomach." No need for port or brandy or whisky. A small dose of *Sulphur* or a short course of *Sulphur* in quite a few days will charm away these symptoms.

I recollect a woman some time ago. She had the symptoms I mentioned which I could only extract with great difficulty. All she complained of was "she was so tired," she could not do anything, she had to sit down and rest, her periods had stopped, she was losing weight, her skin was coarse and inclined to look dirty. She was a very energetic woman as a rule; but when I went into her house I noticed how untidy everything was. The whole family had recently moved to a new house, for weeks afterwards that house remained unfinished, as I had seen it the first week after removal, still the unpacked boxes, etc., everywhere. The beds were unmade at 12 o'clock, everything was indescribably dirty and untidy. The children were not properly washed, their clothes were torn. I saw *Sulphur* around me in that house everywhere. So the lady got it, and the change when I saw her some time afterwards was astounding. Curtains up everywhere, new furniture, all the boxes had disappeared, the beds were made, the linen was clean, the personal cleanliness of mother's children was beyond reproach. And the woman had got buxom again, clear red cheeks, no complaints of tiredness, a general feeling of comfort and well-being in the house.

Sulphur is a great friend to the over-taxed, over-tired women in the forties.

Now do not run away with the idea that *Sulphur* is the only remedy for the menopause, no greater mistake could be made than this. The individual has to be considered in this trouble as well as in any other complaint. I shall illustrate this remark by cases. A certain lady was giving me her symptoms and, while talking about her sudden outbreaks of hot perspiration in a close, warm room which incommoded her very much, I noticed that her eyes filled with tears and without telling me any more, I knew that her remedy was *Pulsatilla*. I heard from her colleagues at the office that she was irritable and changeable, very touchy, which confirmed my diagnosis. So she duly received her quota of *Pulsatilla* with excellent results; her temper became sweeter, her sweats ceased, and her general health improved vastly in quite a short time, to everybody's delight. "She is much easier to get on with" I was told. Homœopathy is a very good "temper" medicine, which I have proved both to myself and to others. For example, a little girl who had been receiving some pills from me for some malady which had made her very irritable, seeing her father in an outburst of rage, fetched her box of pills and presented her father, "Daddy, have one of my pills, they always make me feel good tempered." But we are not talking of bad temper, so we had better return to our subject.

Another time a middle-aged lady was consulting me about her violent headaches, a terrible feeling as if the top of her head was torn off; she was very jumpy, very hysterical, drove her husband to distraction by her fidgets, both day and night; at nights whichever side she lay on, began to twitch, thus preventing sleep. The muscles at the back of the neck were so sore and bruised that the head was drawn back stiffly. Friends had advised osteopathic treatment; well, I could not see anything wrong with her spine; she was assured that her nerves would soon be a thing of the past, that her headaches would disappear, and her rheumatism would no more trouble her; she received *Cimicifuga*, an American plant, and again rapidly she got well, greatly to my relief, for at first she always had such a lot to say, I could never get rid of her, she calmed down so wonderfully that she had very little to say about herself, all her little fads and fancies had evaporated into the blue. At first she strongly reminded me of another remedy, namely, *Lachesis*, which is also a "talking" drug, but the headaches were totally different. The character of the rheumatic pains was so distinctive of *Cimicifuga* that in this case it could not be anything else.

Now that I have mentioned *Lachesis*, we might just as well go on with it, for it is one of the most frequently indicated drugs in troubles of the change of life. Now a person requiring *Lachesis* is very characteristic. One meets them so often in all kinds of women's complaints which are normally very slow to cure, that one is very sorry that orthodox medicine does not know of it and never is likely to know it, unless an enterprising drug manufacturer hears of it and starts to put it on the market with a double-barrelled name attached to it. In the meantime, let ordinary doctors sneer as much as they like and say *Lachesis* or snake poison—it is derived from a South American rattlesnake—can do no good or possibly no harm, as it is digested by the gastric juices, especially when taken in such small doses, as we give it. The people who have been cured by it of their ills would gladly testify to its efficacy, were they asked to do so.

Let me give you an example or two: early last September I noticed that the mother of one of my little patients was very white and drawn, she acknowledged having a severe headache, to which she was subject every ten days or so; they came over her in waves, beginning at the back and passing over to the front of the head, along with it she had distressing palpitations of the heart and pulsations of the body. There was no need to go into further details. I knew what she required.

Now did I give her a dose of headache powder as any orthodox doctor would have done, or a nurse, or for that, any chemist or even most lay people, so much has this evil and pernicious habit of self-drugging penetrated into all circles? No, this woman received the indicated remedy. She was given one powder of *Lachesis* 30, she was not told what to expect; for all she knew she had just received a dose of some sort of pain-killer. I saw her again in a month's time. The change was most striking, she smiled at me and explained that she had had no headaches since her previous visit, an unknown pleasure for years, something which had never happened after taking aspirin. She had been troubled with these heads for years, and they had got steadily worse, and now that the change had started, they had almost become unbearable. She received another dose of *Lachesis* about six weeks after the first, for a slight return of the symptoms; that was four months ago. I see her at regular intervals, there has been no return of the headaches, the palpitations have ceased, the sleep is undisturbed as well, the woman herself looks years younger.

Coincidence, you say, the headaches would have stopped anyhow, they often do when the menses cease. Granted—but the monthlies have become more regular again, altogether she has taken on a new lease of life. Have you ever seen this happen after a course of aspirin? If you are honest, you will agree with me that aspirin only removes the headache temporarily by suppressing the pain, the headache or any other pain for that which you take aspirin always comes back, and you have to take stronger and stronger doses, in the end finishing off by changing over to more powerful anodynes or pain removers. You never see the bloom of youth return to a middle-aged woman—without the artificial aid of cosmetics, mind you—after pain-killers; but you do see this wonder occur before your very eyes again and again, after a properly-indicated remedy has been taken.

However, this is not a lecture on beauty-surgery; so we had better *revenons à nos moutons,* as our friends across the Channel say.

As we are on the subject of headaches during the change of life, my mind recalls another victim of this distressing complaint of the "foolish forties." She had very exacting work to do which demanded close mental application. One hot summer she was extremely bothered with bursting headaches, which she described to me as follows: "Surging pulsations and hammering of the head, nearly driving her frantic, much worse in the warm room and the heat of the sun, relieved by opening the window, cannot lie down in bed, has to sit up in bed in order to get any sleep at all." She got very scared, too, by attacks of palpitations on going up hill. *Glonoin* or *Trinitrin* covered all these alarming symptoms and speedily enabled her to face her long columns of figures with renewed energy. These menopausal disturbances may require any one of the more common remedies; a choice of some forty odd drugs is mentioned in the large repertories under the rubric "Menopause" alone, and that does not include all the medicines, you may have to study in order to really and truly cure the individual.

Now let us tackle another very common and even more crippling and most alarming symptom, namely, hæmorrhage. The orthodox medical profession has very little to offer in the way of treatment for these unfortunate sufferers. The American Eclectic school who are practically unknown in this country, have various herbal remedies for vicarious and excessive bleeding, and so has the common or garden herbalist: but the medical drug cupboard is particularly bare in this respect.

Alas! that the majority of the medical practitioners, even in these enlightened days do not wish to hear about Homœopathy, but condemn it unheard. The mere name Homœopathy is like a red rag to a bull to most of them, and thus they miss many opportunities of curing maladies which they declare incurable, except by the knife. Now this is the typical sequence of events: a professional woman depending on her own earnings to keep herself, was seriously incapacitated by what is technically called Menorrhagia. For a long time she was dosed with ergot, nearly the only remedy the orthodox practitioners know for hæmorrhage. When this was found to be less than useless, she was handed over to the surgeon, and he curetted her first. Later the trouble still persisting, she was placed on the operating table again and robbed of most of her reproductive organs. She was ill for months after this, recuperating from this cruel and quite unnecessary shock to her constitution.

If this woman had been under the care of a homœopathic physician, she would have been saved endless expense, suffering, and her health would have been a hundredfold better. An extravagant claim, you say—yes, maybe—but the homœopathic literature is full of more marvellous cures than this comparatively simple one of curing and stopping hæmorrhages. There are twenty-two remedies given in the repertory under: "Hæmorrhages in the Climacteric Period," and most of them work in record time, provided the patient is willing to give her co-operation and allows the doctor to take a full history of her symptoms. The minutest details are essential and, as I said before, a cure can be guaranteed. Any of the remedies already mentioned may be needed. The menorrhagic patient may require *Sulphur*, and then you would find *Sulphur* symptoms. Or she may need *Lachesis*, and then she would present you with *Lachesis* symptoms.

A long time ago, I met a *Lachesis* patient with a hæmorrhagic history. She had a lot to say for herself, like all the *Lachesis* individuals, she had the bursting heads I have already described, she was hypersensitive to touch, the face was somewhat mottled, she suffered from the heat, suffocated in a warm room, and the uterine hæmorrhage was dark, almost black. All her symptoms would clear up with the hæmorrhage, that is, the day she would be losing, she would be free from headache; the next day she had her headache, but no hæmorrhage. So she was miserable the whole time. After a few short weeks on *Lachesis*, her tale had changed to a jubilate; she took up her old life and her old duties with renewed zest, she had been practically an invalid for a long time past. And the cost to her was negligible, no expensive operation, no prolonged convalescence. How much more preferable, do you not think so?

I have not mentioned a *Sepia* patient so far, which is somewhat remiss of me, as *Sepia* is so often indicated in women's complaints. The uterine hæmorrhage is generally associated with prolapse of the organ, down-bearing pains; they are usually tall, thin people, easily depressed, cold and frigid and spiteful, tired of affection, disliking sympathy. You see women like this almost every day in every walk of life. With it all they have a peculiar complexion, a sallowness, a yellowish-brown discoloration on the face and a yellow saddle, as it is described in the Materia Medica books, across the nose. If you meet such a woman, you can bet your bottom dollar that she wants a dose of *Sepia*, and that *Sepia* will put an end to all her sufferings. I, for one, should not like to be without Sepia. It does valiant work for us women, young or old.

We must not forget *Calcarea carbonica* either. You did not know that lime was a valuable ally to the homœopathic physician, did you? *Calcarea carbonica* women are pale, flabby folk, relaxed and cold, and reserved. Usually they have been busy people who have become tired through overwork. One calls to mind several people suffering from heavy and continuous hæmorrhages during the change, and hardly anybody bleeds as much as a patient who needs *Calcarea carbonica*. Their symptoms point to *Calcarea carbonica*. When they receive a few doses of lime, they lose their chalky look and their muscles firm up all round, the hæmorrhage eases up, too, and there is no need to trouble the surgeon.

At the present moment I have another patient who has been cured without surgery. Her remedy was, and still is, *Nux vomica*. She has been bleeding profusely, just a continual ooze, she was very sensitive to her surroundings, very irritable, in fact, irascible; always quarrelling with her colleagues, terribly easily offended; she felt the cold so much and disliked a draught of air; as for her dyspepsia, that was quite a curse to her, it was always with her, severe pain about an hour after food, always taking things for constipation. A short course of *Nux vomica*, and she became sweeter tempered, and the bleeding was gone. You see, it is quite easy to recognize the *Nux* patient.

There are several other remedies, which might be called for during the climacteric hæmorrhages, such as *Sabina*. In *Sabina* cases the blood is bright red, they have got violent pains shooting up from the sacrum to the front or from the fork upwards to the navel; if you get a woman with these pains and the bright red fluid blood, instead of giving ergot, as is the routine, try a few doses of *Sabina*, and you will be surprised how soon the bleeding will stop. In fact the patient will probably think that it stopped on its own account. *Sabina* is an acute remedy, and if the hæmorrhage recurs again and again, you will require what is called a chronic drug, such as *Sulphur, Calcarea,* etc., according to the symptoms.

The climacteric woman who requires *Crocus* has quite different symptoms. She is rather hysterical, has hæmorrhages with dark clots, and a feeling of weight in the lower part of her abdomen so strongly marked that she is certain that she is about to become a mother, and nothing that you or any other doctor can say, will convince her that this is not so. "But, doctor, I feel the baby move." One mother booked with the nurse in spite of all I said to persuade her to the contrary. We even had a bet on the happy event coming off. I promised her £5 if the baby was born at the time she stated it was due; so certain was I that I was right. She had some few doses of *Crocus*, and she forgot her previous delusion and countermanded the nurse.

Another woman with identical ideas went on for two years

trying to persuade various hospitals in her neighbourhood that she was pregnant. In the end she gave up the unequal contest and put her head in the gas oven. I was grieved, but she was not my patient. Homœopathy would have saved her life. In a case like this the non-treating homœpathic doctor is at a great disadvantage. He must stand by and can say nothing; the lay person can speak up and advise different treatment and change of doctors.

We have a choice of remedies for bleeding during the change. We are not restricted to only one drug, such as ergot, as the allopaths, and when this fails, as it so often does, nothing remains but to advise an operation. And the poor woman is mutilated unnecessarily and suffers endless pain. How much better is the way of the true healer who depends on medicines, herbs of the field in some cases; in others, on metals or salts of metals which are given according to a definite law, and which very rarely let you down, and then it is generally due to not being able to find the right drug. In such a case apply to another authority whose knowledge of drugs is greater than your own, and combined efforts will often achieve the apparently impossible. Only in cases of absolute emergencies should a surgeon be sent for.

TUMOURS

A SURGEON laughed at the idea that a small pea-like cyst of the tongue could be removed by means of medicines; yet he was treading on dangerous ground, for tumours are visible to the eye and palpable to the touch, and are therefore objective and their medicinal removal cannot be laughed out of court, as "faith cures" or the disappearance of merely subjective symptoms, such as you find in rheumatism and other diseases. Is it not curious that a man who stands in awe of the power which a minute organism such as a bacillus typhosus or streptococcus possesses and who fears the power of an ultramicroscopic virus which is said to be the cause of measles and whooping cough, despises and disbelieves in the potency of an attenuated remedy over a mere tumour? "There are more things in heaven and earth, Horatius, than are dreamt of in your philosophy."

There is an old tale which is known to Homœopaths, and it will bear re-telling, a veritable "sermon in stones"—which proves the truth of our law that like cures like. Here it is. A certain Dr. Garth Wilkinson went to Iceland, and he noticed that animals grazing on pastures which were covered with the fine ashes from the lava of Mount Hecla, suffered from enormous bony tumours of the jaw. He brought some of the ashes back to England, triturated it, made it into pills and used it to cure exostosis and other bony tumours, both in horses and human beings. Dr. Burnett and several other homœopathic physicians followed his example, and since that time Hecla lava, as it is still called, is a commonly used remedy for certain types of spongy, bony tumours, which disappear very rapidly under its use. It is more frequently employed in the lower potencies, such as the third decimal, that is 1/1,000 grain doses, or second centesimal triturations, i.e., in 1/10,000 grain doses. I had an interesting case several years back; a woman in the fifties presented herself with a very hard tumour of the kidney. She was sent to a surgeon who removed it and sent her out cured. Twelve months later she came back with a recurrence of the disease, again sent to the surgeon who refused to operate and put her straight on enormous doses of morphia, because of the great pain she suffered from, which became so acute that quite appreciable doses of morphia did not relieve it. She came back and asked: could not something more be done for her? So one was led, rather late in the day, to try what homœopathy could do. She was put on *Hecla lava* 3x, three times a day, and was taken off the morphia, and the *Hecla lava* absolutely removed the pain. The woman had the typical malignant look, a wasted, pallid, exhausted wreck. She picked up in the most astonishing manner, her pallor disappeared, her weakness went, and she started to take up her household duties again, went so far as to do the household washing, and even washed the blankets herself; the tumour became smaller and smaller. The surgeon originally had only given her three months to live. Fifteen months later I sent her back to him, still alive, and with only a trace of the tumour left. Unfortunately she drifted away then; she ceased attending, and one does not know what became of her. Anyway for fifteen months she never had any pain, her tumour had practically disappeared, and she considered herself well enough to go back to her duties. It is not a perfect case, as one does not know the end. But one *does* know the *Hecla lava* relieved, where morphia did not touch it.

I recall another woman who was a circus rider, in the late thirties. She came with a stony, hard swelling in her right breast, the size of a child's head. *Conium maculatum* has the power to produce such hard tumours on the breast, therefore can and does cure as well. She was given *Conium*, or Hemlock, which is its popular name; one does not remember in what potency, but I think it was in the thirtieth potency; and after four months treatment, the hard swelling in the right breast had disappeared. Was it only a mastitis? One had felt tumours of the breast before, and the hardness of an ordinary mastitis was nothing like this stony hardness of this swelling. A stony, hard swelling is usually considered typical of cancer. And yet it disappeared! She came back a year later, and there had been no return!

Then there was a spinster in the early forties, thin and acid; she was very worried about a swelling in her left breast, the size of a tangerine orange. It might have been a cyst only; anyway I tried her on *Phytolacca,* the Poke berry, in the 30th, and later on in the 900th and the 1,000th dilutions, and also ordered compresses of *Phytolacca* mother tincture, to be applied externally every night. She was under treatment for about six months and the swelling, whether only mastitis or malignant cyst, disappeared completely. I saw her five years later, and there had been no return.

I had another lady, who was nearer fifty than forty. She also was very much scared by a "lump" in her left breast, which was tender, and there were also enlarged glands in the left axilla. *Phytolacca* 6 three times a day, and *Phytolacca* compresses, removed this lump and the glands and all her fears. This is now four or five years ago, and she has not had an operation yet!

There was a fourth lady, also unmarried, with a definite lump in her left breast, attached to the nipple, which was retracted. There was a chain of glands extending to the left axilla and a mass of glands palpable in the axilla. She had the usual *Phytolacca*. It has a specific action on the breast; it is an "organ remedy," as Burnett calls it—and again six months later, I searched in vain for any signs of a tumour or glands.

Of course all these cases might have been cases of innocent cysts—non-cancerous growths—I did not incise to find out the nature of the growth—I was content with the fact that they disappeared under the action of the indicated remedy. Years ago I had another case, a poor, hard-working widow woman, just an office cleaner, but such a nice creature, a natural lady. She came to me with an enormous malignant cancer of her breast. I blame myself to this day and cannot forgive myself for telling her that she had cancer. She went to the surgeon, who removed it, but she would not make an effort and in less than nine months later she died of recurrence in the spine, in terrible agony. Poor dear, she came too late, and I did not then know enough of the power of the homœopathic remedy which, when it cannot cure, can and does remove pain, so that a patient has a peaceful end. Morphia stupefies and dulls a patient; it is said to be kind to give morphia, but one finds that with our remedies, morphia is not needed. It is surprising how peaceful a person is under homœopathic medicines.

Now for some examples of cures of simple tumours under our treatment. Some four years ago a young man turned up with multiple wens of the scalp. He had them removed by a surgeon on at least two different occasions; but they always came back. I removed two growths for him, one the size of a large bean and the other the size of a walnut; then I gave him *Graphites* 1 m, and he kept on it for some time. He has had no return of the wens since then. This, of course, might only be a coincidence again; but it is a well-recognized fact that *Graphites* acts on wens and prevents their recurrence.

I had a run of Meibomian cysts lately. These are small cysts of the upper eyelid, and the usual treatment advised is removal by the knife. A friend in the fifties developed such a cyst in her left upper eyelid, which came up almost in a night and grew so rapidly that her left eye was nearly closed up. I advised her to go and see an eye surgeon about its removal, and she threw down the gauntlet to me and asked "Cannot some of your wonderful remedies cure this cyst without an operation?" I hesitated and admitted it might be possible, but it would take longer than the surgeon's treatment. He could do it in a few minutes, while the homœopathic remedy would require days and weeks. I remembered, she had been vaccinated several times, she bore huge ugly marks on her arms, and the last once or twice the vaccination had not taken. Here was a clue. This might be a case of vaccinosis, which, as Dr. Burnett claimed, often produces cysts as a late manifestation. It was worth trying anyway to give *Thuja* as an antidote. It was a left-sided cyst, the patient was never at her best in the early mornings, never woke up until the day was well aired; and the history of repeated vaccinations; here was the three-legged stool, upon which to base the homœopathic prescription. And it worked. Instead of growing bigger and closing up the eye completely, as the cyst had threatened to do, after *Thuja* 30 had been given, it began to shrink imperceptibly, and without any pain or discomfort it disappeared without leaving any trace. It was "spurlos versenkt" indeed, swallowed up by the action of the *Thuja*. And this patient in the process of a cure developed an irritating eruption on her feet, first on the inside of the arches of the feet, which spread all over the soles, and then this eruption crept up to the ankles. She was very much tried by this skin trouble which itched and burnt and burnt and itched, whenever she sat near the fire or took her stockings off, and the agony of the nights! The moment the feet got warm, she was wakened by this irritation and had to sit up half the night, scratching her feet. In the end, in order to be comfortable and get some sleep, she had to hang her feet out of bed, and every night the bed had to be remade in this manner, so that the sheets and blankets only went as far as the ankles. This cure therefore proceeded in the correct homœopathic manner : the cure took place from within outwards; the particular toxin, in this case the vaccinosis, was eliminated through the skin. The lady was wise in the lore of Homœopathy, she did not apply any external remedies, any lotions or ointments to drive in the external manifestation of the disease, but asked for a remedy to cure this dermatitis. I gave *Sulphur* 30, on : irritation worse heat, worse undressing, better hanging feet out of bed; but there was no change; the condition remained the same. On further study of the symptoms, I realised that I had overlooked certain characteristics : the patient carefully removed all fat from the meat, she was touchy and irritable, liked sympathy; this along with her great aversion to heat and exhaustion, and general aggravation of all her symptoms from heat, completed the picture of *Pulsatilla*, and *Puls*, in high potencies, 30th potency, and later in the 1*m*, cleared up the skin eruption.

The cure took several weeks, as I predicted; but it was well worth while, as a surgeon would have removed only the foreign body, the cyst, the external manifestation of the internal disease. The actual trouble, the internal disease, which produced the cyst, would still be there. Homœopathy removed not only the external manifestations, but also the internal disease by eliminating it via the skin; and another remedy—*Pulsatilla* to wit—took up the cure and finished it.

Much about the same time I came across another case of Meibomian cyst, a woman in the thirties who had this swelling for months. It did not worry her, except for cosmetic reasons. I gave her a note to the Eye Hospital to have it removed. Somehow she was busy, and she never went to the hospital. I was forced, therefore, to try what medicines could do. There was a history of tuberculosis in the family; she was thin, had a tendency to colds and coughs, felt the cold very much—therefore I started her on *Tuberculinum* 30 in weekly doses. For the frequent nasal catarrhs and slight feverish chills, which troubled her so often, I gave various remedies, as required. *Pulsatilla* in repeated doses during one feverish attack; *Bryonia* 30 three times daily for a persistent dry cough with pain behind the sternum and great thirst, during a later attack. She told me she usually kept this cough all through the winter. *Bryonia* considerably modified the bronchial catarrh, but not completely. On further enquiry I discovered that she was an inveterate smoker; she smoked over forty cigarettes a day and only had one good meal, the cigarettes served instead of a meal. Naturally she was suffering from chronic tobacco poisoning, which had to be antidoted. There is one drug which not only antidotes tobacco, but also stops the craving for it; this is *Caladium*, a South American Arum—and on reading up this remedy in the Materia Medica, I found the mental characteristics of this patient, the forgetfulness and the absentmindedness, the things that were put in the wrong places, and were lost; the nervous excitement; always in a hurry and scurry—everything was done in great haste; she was always flying about. I chose *Caladium* 6, and she was asked to take it every night and morning—and, strange to relate, she told me a week or two later, she did not enjoy smoking any more, she could only smoke three or four cigarettes a day, instead of forty or fifty. The cysts, there were two small cysts on the upper eyelid, have disappeared, in time the nervous symptoms ought to disappear as well. The cure of these cysts has taken about six months —a very slow process, perhaps, but the whole patient is being treated, and such constitutional treatment is lengthy, sometimes.

Now for case No. 3. This is a middle-aged lady, who was vaccinated a good many times and had not "taken" the last twice. On that indication she was given *Thuja* 30, and she is getting rid of her cysts beautifully in record time. She has taken *Thuja* now for about six weeks, and one cannot see the swelling any more. So far there have been no untoward symptoms, such as skin eruptions, or such-like unpleasant things. They do not follow always after homœopathic medication, and cures take place without subsequent external manifestations. The point to remember is, if and when skin eruptions follow while taking remedies, do not suppress these by applying external lotions and ointments, but let your physician know; he will treat this eruption with medicines and cure it from within.

These are just a few examples of the power of the correctly indicated remedy over such external manifestations of internal disease, as tumours. Our literature is full of examples of cures of cysts and other tumours by means of medicines : Carleton in his *Homœopathy in Medicine and Surgery*, gives a few examples. Burnett in various booklets gives more examples. What has been done in the past, can still be done today. Therefore, as Burnett says : "Machs nach, und machs besser," i.e., "Imitation is the best form of flattery," and "Try to improve on it," if you can.

COLITIS

Many years ago I saw a pathetic letter in a well-known medical magazine, in which an elderly doctor appealed to his colleagues for suggestions how to cure his colitis which had been troubling him for years and was now incapacitating him entirely. Physician, heal thyself, I thought. What a confession of ignorance! I carefully scanned the journal in question for weeks after to see whether the poor old doctor got any help. But the answers were few and far between, and most of them very discouraging. They were mainly from fellow sufferers, who all complained that they had tried all and sundry things with but little success. I was still too young and diffident, and to this day I reproach myself for not having stretched out a helping hand; for Homœopathy has many remedies for colitis, one need never despair. It has been my luck to have had some colitis cases lately, and for the help of other victims I pass on the glad tidings.

I had watched a poor young woman for a year or two, seeing her steadily getting thinner and paler; she was under hospital treatment, and I could do nothing. It was a pitiful story, husband out of work for years, seven children, the man had run out of benefit, the whole family on relief, the mother always going short, in order to make the food go further for the little ones, result of this under-feeding was colitis. Hers was a tale of a song of sixpence, or a lack of them.

One day she was full to overflowing about her own burden; if she was only well enough to work, to earn a few more shillings to augment her tiny income; but she could not drag herself about at all. She was hurried out of bed every day of her life at 5 o'clock by the urgent call of nature; she had to fly in order to get there in time, and then she passed pints of white jelly. This went on all the morning. So it was not safe for her to go out until the afternoon, and the pain was terrific; and then there was blood as well, basins full, no wonder she was miserable. And the medicine the hospital gave her made her so much worse, she moaned, she suffered agonies after it. The lady-almoner had tried to console her by telling her of a friend of hers who also had colitis for years, and the only relief she ever had was from some patent medicine she got from some quack. Fancy an almoner of a hospital so far forgetting herself as to recommend some quack's rubbish for a patient and to give her doctors away by saying that nothing could cure colitis! A fine state of affairs, and yet not to be wondered at; for there is nothing in orthodox medicine for colitis, or there is such a plethora of recommendations. Each man has a different idea of how to set about to cure it, that one knows it has beaten the doctor. One man advises one variety of injections, another man something totally different, and the third sings the praises of yet something quite different, and the honest doctor shrugs his shoulders and won't advise anything.

Well, to go on with my tale, I turned to the woman and bluntly asked her, "Why go on with the hospital medicine if it does not do you any good and makes you so much worse?" She was stumped, she could not answer me, so I rashly offered to cure her, if she would put herself under my care for some time. She hesitated, so I bribed her with the offer of invalid dinners, and more for the sake of the free gift of the dinners, she gave in and promised to swallow my stuff, with very little faith; for, like most poor people, she had hospitalitis very badly. These people, as a rule, take the word of any young whippersnapper of a house-surgeon before the advice of an experienced doctor in general practice.

I went home, nearly tearing my hair that I had given her my word to cure her, when I saw the many common* symptoms I had got out of her. On looking them up in the *Repertory*, it might have been one of several drugs. The symptoms strongly suggested Sulphur to me, but *Hydrastis* had the passing of copious, white slime as well, and there were a few other drugs. I plumped for Sulphur on this symptom: Rushing out of bed in the early morning. At any rate it would clear the deck, and bring forth other distinctive symptoms, taking into consideration the variety of strong stuff she had taken from the hospital. I gave her *Sulphur* 30, hoping for the best, and also had her weighed. She had lost well over 2 stones during the last year. No particular instructions could be given about her diet. It was just a matter of Hobson's choice. She had to eat what she could get, except in

* N.B.—Common symptoms mean: symptoms common to and always found in that particular disease.

the middle of the day, when I ordered her a milk and egg diet.

The results surpassed my wildest hopes. She put on half a pound in the first week, the diarrhœa improved, the slime almost ceased at once, and a fortnight later she reported that her bowels only moved four times a day instead of a dozen times. The pain was greatly relieved, so I left well alone.

In six weeks she had gained 4 pounds. A month later she presented herself again with another jubilate; no diarrhœa, no colitis, no pain, and gain of over 8 pounds. In March, a short four months after starting the treatment, there was a slight return of the bleeding on a normal diet or lack of diet; so a dose of *Sulphur* 1*m.* was handed to her. In May, a return of colitis, after some teeth had been extracted under a general anæsthetic—mind you, the teeth were extracted when the diarrhœa had cleared up. She received *Sulphur* 6 night and morning for a week. The brave woman had been to work since early January, as soon as she felt well enough. There was no slackness with her. So you see, a woman who had been ill for over thirteen months with colitis and hæmorrhages, and had lost well on 2 stones in that time under ordinary medical treatment, got cured in a few short weeks without any dieting, and without any effort on her part.

Another case. Here I did not know even that the lady in question had colitis. She was of the old school, who did not mention such an indelicate subject as her internal organs. She had been in the tropics, had swallowed much quinine, had had dysentery, and now suffered from goitre; she also had a great deal of rheumatism in her wrist and finger joints, for which she came to me, asking for light treatment. I prescribed *Natrum mur.* rather vaguely as an antidote to over-doses of quinine, first in the 6th centesimal dilution, later *Nat. mur.* was given in the 12th centesimal, repeating it once a day for weeks. Some few months after she confided in me that she had never expected to get rid so completely of her rheumatism, and that the colitis she had been subject to had cleared up miraculously as well. So you see, you do not need to diagnose all the complaints of a patient, you only require to know some symptoms, the most important by preference, and you can cure him or her of all kinds of things the treating doctor knows nothing about at first. Do not run away with the idea that artificial sunlight treatment had very much to do with the cure. She only had light about one day in a fortnight, as she lived out of town and could not come up any oftener. No, it was a case of the little sugar pills again.

Case No. 3. This was a different type of colitis, only seen in babies. It is congenital, existing from birth, and is caused by an enormous dilation of the colon, the large intestine. This is blown up like a balloon, and its contents are discharged downwards, as soon as they enter the small intestines. The miserable infant is in a constant state of running from the bowels, the picture is usually that of a poor thin child, with wasted extremities and large belly. Nothing can be done for it as rule, I have seen four cases of this unpleasant disease. The first died in hospital, after a venturesome surgeon had decided to operate on it! The second is still in hospital and has been there for over three years. The surgeon is waiting, until it is old enough for him to operate, I suppose. He will remove a few yards of bowel and hopes to settle the disease in this fashion. In the meantime the child is still having diarrhœa, is still having an enormous abdomen, poor little thing. The third I lost sight of. Probably it is either dead or leading a miserable existence in some hospital ward, waiting for the surgeon's knife.

When I saw this child first, I had a straight talk with the mother and offered to cure the baby, provided she kept him under my care for months. He was then four months old, weighed 11 pounds, measured 18 inches round his navel; he was terribly distended. He was nearly as broad round his tummy, as he was long, all belly and nothing else. The moment he started taking the breast, his bowels started to run. Quite a hydrant of green watery fluid shot out of his bowel with a great deal of force. In order to save herself from being swamped by this fluid, the mother had to tie the baby on the chamber on her lap.

We tried various remedies with little or no success. Still the bowels acted, as soon as the baby was being fed.

Various friends urged hospital treatment. The mother retained her faith, and her faith was rewarded at last. On October 17th the boy got a dose of *Magnesia carbonica* 30. The abdominal circumference was then 19 inches. Much to the mother's joy the motions were slightly more yellow, did not look like frog's spawn any more. Another dose of the same medicine was given at the end of October. Altogether some half dozen doses of *Carbonate of Magnesia* were dispensed until the middle of February, that is in four months. He has had nothing since, he has never ailed anything, there has never been any trouble with his teeth. At seven months he had his first tooth, at eight months he had six teeth, at eleven months eight teeth, his height was 28 inches. At a year he weighed 22 pounds, and was the proud possessor of ten teeth. And his colitis went gradually. The first time his motions were yellow and firm, his mother rushed to her neighbours to tell them the tidings of great joy. That was at seven months.

At thirteen months he is absolutely the picture of health, robust, rosy, full of life, full of mischief, of course walking for weeks, talking—and no colitis! Where is the congenital dilatation of the colon? Gone where the good niggers go; gone for ever, never to return. Impossible, you will say: I am romancing, to put it mildly. Ask the mother, ask the neighbours, ask the nurse who saw him weekly at the weighing centre, they will tell you the same story. A few simple powders worked the miracle. And thanks be to God who opened the eyes of His servant Hahnemann to show his successors the way they should go to heal the sick by such simple means.

There are various types of colitis. Some are chronic and long-standing, others are very acute and rapidly fatal. I am not going to weary you with scientific descriptions of these varieties, nor with pathological details; but just dip into my bag of memory and recall a few incidents. I was still quite raw, a young medico in her first house-surgeon's job, and we had an elderly man in the ward suffering from ulcerative colitis who was passing quantities of foul pus and blood. The cause of the trouble was unknown. I cannot recall now, what treatment was given him. The senior physicians were puzzled, and nothing could be done. In due course he was gathered to his ancestors, and the unpleasant duty of performing a *post mortem* fell to me. I discovered the site of the lesions and the particular variety of the colitis, but paid for my indiscretion in investigating too closely by being stricken myself with a sharp and painful attack of acute colitis, a temperature of 104, acute diarrhœa, passing much blood and pus.

I had to retire to bed and was given by the visiting doctor some bismuth mixture which duly achieved the desired effect of producing constipation. Then there was total stoppage, and that had to be counteracted by a dose of castor oil. This was the one and only time in my life I have taken castor oil, and that was under protest. I remember, as I proved refractory, and the nurses could not manage to get the stuff down my throat, the august matron herself, appearing at my bedside and mixing the fatal draught, sandwiched between two layers of black coffee, and standing over me, until it had gone down. I admitted it was quite tasteless, but the after-effects! I grumbled: "First you make me constipated, and then you start the diarrhœa again. There does not seem any sense in that treatment." I was ill for about a week, a martyr to my profession, infected in the course of my duties. Doctors run many risks, and most of them do it gladly and cheerfully for the sake of humanity. I had learned my lesson as well: never would I treat a patient in the same way as I had been treated.

Many years later I had another attack of colitis. This time it was the result of eating cherries in Switzerland and drinking ice-cold water straight from the chattering brooklets on long tramps, when overheated and tired. These brooks are sometimes hotbeds of infection through pollution from cattle and herdsman; and you are warned not to drink the water without boiling it. The symptoms were: yellow, watery stools with flatulence, painless, and coming on worse after eating. When taking into consideration the cause of the trouble, namely eating fruit, the remedy was pretty plain. It was *China*. I took *China* 1*m.*, and one dose put me right. There was no subsequent constipation, no need for taking a nauseous draught of castor oil, everything was quite simple and straightforward, much nicer than the orthodox procedure.

A friend who was with me on the same trip also developed colitis. She did not mention it for some time, and tried to cure it herself. She had a good deal of pain, passed quantities of mucous and had many loose motions. She was very much scared by my diagnosis of colitis. What a lot there is in a name! Everybody told her of people they had known who had had colitis for many years. She got quite a phobia about it and, perhaps as a result of it, she did not give her symptoms as clearly as usual. Anyway, we had much trouble in clearing it up. She lost nearly all faith in me.

In the end I had a vaccine made from the secretions, and she was given graduated doses of homœopathic dilutions of the particular bacillus which caused the colitis, not by the painful method of injection, but by the mouth. This I find answers very well, in spite of the derogatory remarks of pathologists, who will not admit that this method of giving vaccines produces any results.

In this case it did the trick—*Bacillus Morgan* in the 30th dilution cleared up the colitis.

A short course was all that was necessary and then the constitutional remedy came in again, and finished the cure. This was *Pulsatilla*. It was interesting how it worked, once the action of the bacillus was antidoted. It would not touch the colitis before.

Each case presents its own problems, and one has to take each patient individually. Just because a particular person has been cured by say, *China*, from colitis, it does not follow that each case of colitis requires *China*. Far from it. There are many different medicines for colitis. It often requires much study and hours of work, before the right remedy is discovered. I have got an old book here by my side, which is called *Bell on Diarrhœa and Dysentery*. There are 150 pages on diarrhœa, and it describes the actions of 108 remedies for this bowel complaint. Colitis is only a comparatively recent term, and one of its symptoms is diarrhœa. The older writers were not so wrapped up in pathological names like the modern product of medical schools. Well, these 108 medicines are not by any means all the drugs that you may have to study, before the right one is found, and you may even have to give a remedy quite outside the range of this book.

I shall give you a case to illustrate this. This patient came to me some time ago for rheumatism in her wrists and palms, not for colitis at all. She had lived in the tropics for a number of years, she was a very prim and proper lady, and such a thing as colitis could not be mentioned. She asked for ultra-violet ray treatment for her pains, and had some treatment at irregular intervals, as she could not come up to town very regularly. In the end, as her rheumatism improved only very slowly, I advised medicinal treatment, and, on her past medical history, which included radium treatment for goitre of the neck, and on the supposition that she had had most likely an overdose of radium which produces rheumatic pains in the hands, I prescribed *Radium bromide*, 12th centesimal dilution. The effects were quite astonishing. The rheumatism cleared up remarkably quickly. She declared she had not felt so well for years, and then she let out that her colitis, which had troubled her for years ever since her stay in India, had disappeared at the same time. So you will see you do not need to know all the pathological ailments which afflict a certain patient, if you prescribe on homœopathic principles, which I did in this case. The large doses of radium had caused the rheumatism. In antidoting the overdoses of radium by minute doses of a well triturated and diluted *Radium*, the disease that was active in the background was cured as well. Very gratifying indeed. This lady had almost identical symptoms with the lady on page 104, who was cured with *Natrum muriaticum*. This antidoted the quinine that had been given previously, and at the same time dealt with the rest of the various ailments, the rheumatism and the colitis. If this *Natrum muriaticum* had been given years ago the goitre would have cleared up as well; one has seen many cases of goitre cured by medicines alone, not necessarily *Natrum muriaticum* always. Other remedies may be indicated.

Now another case, where I have not been so successful. It was full of complications. The lower classes, when asked what a certain relative died of are very fond of mysteriously telling you that he or she died of "complications", which means several pathological diseases in one person. This was such a case of "complications". The good lady certainly had some crosses to bear. She had lupus of the face and nose and eyes, there were gastritis and colitis and occasional attacks of phlebitis, and she was cursed with an incurably artistic temperament. She was always late and behind in everything; full of excuses for her faults, lively and interesting in the evening, but not the slightest bit of use in the morning. She was a typical tubercular individual, long and lanky and cadaverous. You wondered how long she was going to last, whether the next spell of cold weather would finish her, as the winter shrivelled her to nothing. Yet, like a bad penny, she always turned up again and, like Micawber, she always had some new ideas of making money and kept you interested in her ideas and plans. Poor thing, what an inheritance.

We tried many things for her various complaints. I gave her *Lachesis* once for her colitis, as the stools were offensive, and diarrhœa alternated with constipation, and she was worse in the spring and afflicted me badly with her loquacity. *Lachesis* brought out an alarming attack of purpura on the lower extremities, first on the left and then on the right leg, and agonizing pain. I had to send her to bed for six weeks, which improved the general condition. Then she left town on one of her periodic disappearing tricks, and I heard nothing of her for months.

On her return she presented the following symptoms: diarrhœa after fruit and coffee, irresistible urging to stool very early

in the morning; then there were catarrhal symptoms, thick yellow
mucus in the nose and eyes, with a burning feeling in the nose.
So she got *Cistus canadensis*, a medicine which has all the tubercular eruptions in its make-up. My friend was extremely sensitive
to all medicines. She promptly got another aggravation which
took the form of an acute catarrh with a rise of temperature.
Once more bed for her, but not so long this time. It will take
time before she is cured of her inherited disease. If only she would
keep under treatment, one could do more for her. Unfortunately
she suffers also from an overdose of pride and a lack of £ s. d.,
a bad combination.

N.B.—This lady kept away from me for financial reasons for
two years, then tried to get in touch with me while I was away
on holidays. Not finding me, she went to hospital for her latest
complaint : a small tumour of the breast. This I heard about six
months later. Alas, she had so much radium by that time that
nothing could be done for her. She died in hospital.

An old lady rises before my mind's eye. She came to me with
a fractured humerus and a long tale of woe of it having been
badly set in hospital—it was during the war, and the hospitals
were run by dressers, and the civilians were neglected in the
general mad rush of the more serious war casualties. The arm
was not in alignment at all and had to be set all over again. The
plucky old dame was very brave over it too, and the pain was
much relieved by the homœopathic pain-killer, *Arnica*. She
fondly imagined she was getting morphia, and I did not enlighten her. On getting her better, I discovered that, as a result
of years of suffering from colitis, she had gradually cut down her
diet so that she lived on brown bread and Ivelcon cheese. Fruit,
eggs, vegetables, everything gave her pain and diarrhœa. So
gradually I changed the *Arnica* powders to *Sulphur* which has
this aversion to all sorts of articles of food strongly marked. Also
this good lady loved arguments. She was fond of philosophical
and metaphysical arguments. So *Sulphur* was the choice. After
about two months' treatment, I gently suggested, she should try
various other additions to her menu. She was rather doubtful,
but carried out orders and found to her joy that the colitis had
gone, while the broken arm was mending. "Granny is not
peculiar any more," confided her little grandchild to me.

Then there is that case of rheumatic fever, followed by tuberculosis of the peritoneum. She had one foot in the grave, she was

not even a walking skeleton, but just a living bag of bones. Only her brave smile told you she was still alive, and determined to carry on in spite of priests, specialists and fidgety relatives. The terrible weakness with the marked emaciation put me on the track of the right remedy. It was *Selenium*, a rare metal, used in dictaphones and sensitive plates of electrical burglar alarms, which made a sound healthy woman out of one who was given up by everybody. She was alive fifteen years later, without a trace of heart disease or any other weakness, and able to work hard at her church work. A living memorial to the power of Homœopathy.

I found out afterwards that she had had bouts of colitis for more than twenty years previously, unable to eat apples, oranges or lemons, unless she wished to produce days of suffering and diarrhœa. After she got up from her bed of sickness, which so nearly became her deathbed, all signs of or tendency to colitis disappeared, and she could indulge in fruit, as much as she liked. If she had had *Selenium* twenty years before, she would never have had that fatal abdominal weakness, which helped in giving her tubercular peritonitis! If only the general public knew, and the medical profession did not scorn Homœopathy, how much less suffering there would be in this vale of tears!

Now in conclusion, just a few words about how to take a case of, and how to report on, a case of colitis. Notice carefully the nature of the motions, their consistency, their colour; whether blood, slime or just watery stuff is present; whether they are painless or not, whether they are scanty or the reverse, contain undigested food; involuntary or not, whether odourless or fœtid. What ameliorates the stools, warmth or cold, pressure or bending over or stretching; what aggravates them, what foods, eating, drinking, whether day or night, walking or resting brings on the diarrhœa. What are the sensations before, during and after stools. Take note of any other symptoms that accompany the motions, restlessness, flatulence, much thirst, desire for anything out of the ordinary. Is there any vomiting? The more closely you watch each attack, and the more detailed the symptoms are, the sooner you will be cured of this chronic and weakening complaint, provided you go to a good Homœopath who has studied his Materia Medica and knows his drugs. And do not fall into the fatal error of cutting down your diet and only living on one or two foodstuffs. The more you limit your meals, and the less variety you have, the more chronic your complaint will become. You will find that after some time on homœopathic treatment you will be able to eat and digest many things you could not look at before. But do not expect miracles to happen in a day or two. Give the medicines time to act.

SOME ACUTE CASES

(1) WAKENED by loud ringing of telephone about 3 a.m. Agitated voice at the other end of the wire reporting feeling extremely ill, with sensation of impending death, shaking and trembling of muscles—one could hear the chattering of the teeth and the shaking of the telephone—there was heat of the body, much heat of the lower extremities. No cause could be given for this sudden attack, which roused the patient from a deep sleep. Ptomaine poisoning was considered, but, even though mushrooms had been partaken of the previous night, the other members of the family were not struck down : there was no vomiting or diarrhœa. The remedy lay between *Aconite* and *Arsenic*; but *Aconite* won the day, as one remembered the suddenness of the attack, the fact that the patient was a plethoric, strong, well-developed indivi- dual, somewhat choleric—and the day before had been cold, dry, and somewhat windy. *Aconite* 30 was prescribed over the telephone, to be taken at 10 to 15 minutes' interval. Result : no further disturbance during the night; patient went to sleep in about two hours' time and was able to go to work by 8.30 in the morning, none the worse for this unpleasant experience. Patho- logical diagnosis was impossible and unnecessary, as diagnosis of the required indicated remedy was immediate, and the disease process was cut short.

(2) Another nocturnal dénouement. Patient suddenly wakened shortly after midnight by acute abdominal colic and nausea, could hardly get out of bed quick enough in order to get to the lavatory with simultaneous explosion at both ends. Vomiting of extremely bitter bile and loose, very offensive diarrhœa : it was as if a tap was turned on, and there was no holding back. This happened two or three times, accompanied with great prostra- tion, restlessness and anguish, and a feeling as if the end was near. *Arsenic* 1m. given and repeated two or three times at short intervals, and the attack ceased as suddenly as it came on, thanks to the efficiency of the correctly given medicine. The choice of

the remedy was made easy, as it was remembered that the previous afternoon at a well-known restaurant, ice-cream and cream cakes had been on the menu; and diarrhœa after ice-cream points to *Arsenic*. There was no recurrence of this acute gastroenteritis. The patient wisely starved for twenty-four hours in order to give the inflamed mucous membranes of the stomach and intestines a good rest.

(3) Called out before 8 a.m. Found young woman writhing in bed with acute abdominal colic and stitching, burning pains; the pains were so severe she wanted to move, but every movement made her shriek out; she had to lie still with the knees drawn up to relax the abdominal muscles; she did not want to be touched, every breath she took made her pain worse. She was asking for cold water, which she would gulp down in big mouthfuls. They were newly married, and the poor husband stood by holding her hand, absolutely helpless and worked up. On examination, one found the typical signs of an acute appendicitis: the attack had come on during the early hours of the night; the temperature was 100°, pulse 100-110. One wondered about operation and admitting the patient to hospital, but decided to give Homœopathy a chance. The patient's symptoms called for *Bryonia*, and *Bryonia* 1m, given half-hourly relieved so quickly that after two doses the abdominal muscles relaxed, and by 11 a.m., two hours after she had the first dose, she was sound asleep, the temperature and pulse were normal, and the attack was over. She was seen the next day perfectly recovered, happy and smiling. What a godsend Homœopathy is! The family and the patient were saved the agitation of removal to hospital, the anxiety of a more or less serious operation, followed by several weeks of convalescence, let alone the expense of it all. She was subsequently given a diet sheet, warned about constipation, forbidden to take irritating laxatives, and three years later there had been no return of any acute abdominal trouble.

(4) A young woman, aged 18, came on November 23rd, 1936, complaining of recurrent attacks of gall-bladder colic with jaundice and vomiting: had three attacks since birth of child; attacks every three to four weeks. Said she had never had a day's illness until she became pregnant: jaundice and sickness developed some time before the child was born. She was kept in hospital, as she was so ill; they X-rayed her three times and sent her out with the diagnosis, obstruction of gall-bladder, and with a very

strict diet—no fat, no butter, skimmed milk, fish, etc., to which she stuck religiously, and yet the attacks recurred.

A few more exact symptoms were elicited, such as: pains recurred every night, hammering pains right side region of gall-bladder extending through the right shoulder-blade, restless with pain, sits bent over with pain, has to hold herself. This suggested *Chelidonium*; on the other hand there was a craving for fat (*Ars., Hep., Nit. ac., Nux v.* and *Sulph.*) and a desire for sweets which left *Ars., Nux v.* and *Sulph.*—*Sulphur* being indicated in the highest degree. Mentally she was a *Sulphur* patient too: intelligent, inquisitive, wanted to know the why and wherefore of everything—a typical know-all, argumentative philosopher. *Sulphur* 30 was decided on. A week later the report was: ever so much better, no further attacks of pain or of jaundice.

On December 11th reported that she could not resist a good helping of suet pudding three or four days previously, had some pain and retching for four hours, but attack passed off quickly and there was no jaundice. *Sulphur* 6 night and morning prescribed, as *Sulphur* 30 did not hold long enough. December 21st: no more pains, no jaundice, feeling ever so well in herself, has not felt so well for months, has not had any period, since baby was born, wondered if she was pregnant again. Continued *Sulphur* 6 night and morning.

January 4th, 1937: very well, no further attacks, has been on ordinary diet; the period came on Christmas Day. Wants to know what the medicine was, and wonders why the hospital could not have given her the same, simple pills that cured her so quickly. A *Sulphur* patient is frequently an eternal question mark and wants to probe into everything. Is very grateful for having been saved further lengthy examinations and investigations, and a threatened operation, and insists on taking a further supply of pills with her, so that she can keep them by her in case of another attack.

Corollary. One wonders what would happen if the majority of doctors were Homœopaths! Many acute illnesses would be cut short, there would be less hospital beds required, fewer operations, public money would be saved, and valuable lives would be prolonged. Shall we ever see the day when Homœopathy is preached from the house tops and taught in all the medical schools?

EPILEPSY CURED BY *LYCOPODIUM*

THERE are certain diseases for which orthodox medicine has no cure, or perhaps it were better to say that the so-called cure is worse than the disease; or at best one can only say that the treatment consists in never giving up taking the medicine for the rest of one's life. An example of such an unfortunate sufferer who is condemned to never-ceasing doses of nauseous draughts is an epileptic. The usual advice of the doctor for an epileptic is to write a prescription for a bromide mixture in ever-increasing doses, and what is even worse, since the curse of the group of barbiturate medicines has been discovered, luminal is added to the bromide and the poor afflicted ones become nothing but a storehouse of bromides and luminal. The fits may become suppressed by these remedies, or they may not : sometimes they recur again and again in spite of bromide, and eventually the poor unfortunate one has to be taken into a mental home for epileptics and must needs end his days there, driven there not by the disease, but by the cumulative effects of the bromides. And one has heard that since luminal has been given, that the ratio of admission to mental homes for epileptics has steadily risen. Any brain power that an epileptic ever possessed is steadily undermined and destroyed by the bromides and such like medicines; and yet this is all that the orthodox can offer in the way of alleviation. The more's the pity. Can Homœopathy do any better? It could, if it were given the chance : our literature is full of examples of epilepsy cured by the homœopathic remedy given according to the law of the simillimum. But, alas our old books are out of print, and anyway, are not read by the majority; only a small minority of the medical fraternity are willing to study our system, and apply it.

Under this heading comes a most interesting case of epilepsy which was cured by a remedy given homœopathically; that means it was prescribed because the symptoms, as given by the patient, revealed that a certain medicine was required and *that* medicine cured, so that no further fits or epileptic attacks occurred. No notice was taken of the attack *per se*, or the type of convulsion; but the whole patient was considered, his psychology or mental make-up was carefully studied, and his remedy was found mainly on his mental characteristics, as Kent, of America, taught us.

Now for the history. This young man, aged 27, had been suffering upwards of two years from definite epileptic fits which used to take him unawares going to work, so that he often found himself waking up in the casualty rooms of various hospitals. He was a very strong-minded young man and had ideas of his own, and one of them was : he wished to be treated homœopathically, so he ever steadfastly refused the orthodox draughts offered by the house surgeons, in spite of their scorn that a disease such as his, such as epilepsy was, could be treated by anything but *proper medicine*. He wended his way to the local homœopathic hospital, and also tried a hybrid Homœopath with great faith, but little response. One cannot do very good work in a busy out-patients' department, and it takes time to take the history and details of the symptoms according to Hahnemann, and as it is impossible to devote a very long time, such as an hour, to each patient, it follows that some cases are missed, and the results are not always striking or brilliant. Well, this young man presented the following symptoms : First seen May 20th, 1935; the fits come on after having a good sleep, and at varying intervals, usually has at least one fit a week, the longest interval has been thirty days.

The aura is : "head feels like a balloon and seems to expand; quiver of light in forehead before attacks"; some of his fellow workers told him that they have noticed a small red swelling like a blood blister underneath his left eye which gets larger and more prominent just before he has an attack.

Feels stupid and dazed after fit, bites tongue, and has been told that he is unconscious for ten to twelve minutes. Has a slight headache and feeling of weakness which wears off gradually.

There is also nausea and desire to vomit after an attack, as he usually swallows blood. Has had several attacks during his sleep.

In appearance he is well made, fair skinned, greasy, pimply and blotchy face; very pale and anæmic, complains his face is very tender when he shaves, due to the numerous pimples.

His general symptoms were : gets irritable and annoyed and angry, specially when asked questions which he considers silly; prefers his own company, is better alone; hates sympathy, hates being asked how he is; sullen, then flares up suddenly; likes walking; walks for miles without speaking to anybody; somewhat indifferent to his family; the weather does not affect him except in close thundery conditions; has vertigo, worse rushing about, swaying from left to right; has been vaccinated once; is worse in the afternoon, if awake; cannot take bananas, but has craving for apples.

Advice given : not to take any stimulants, no coffee, no peppermint; put on a strict non-meat diet, advised to live only on fruit, vegetables, raw salads, milk, cheese, eggs.

(I have found from experience that epileptic attacks are kept at bay, if no meat is taken.)

The prescription was : *Lyc.* 6 nightly, largely given on his mental symptoms, those of an obstinate person, with a very logical mind, and somewhat contemptuous of those he considers fools, yet personally lacking in self-confidence.

There were also the time symptoms, the time aggravation in the afternoons. At a later sitting it was elicited that the aggravation was also between 4 to 8 a.m. The curious part about this is that this young man was a night worker, and therefore his 4 to 8 morning aggravation occurred when he had been up for hours and really corresponded to the afternoon aggravation of the ordinary day worker. An interesting point, which was not brought out at the first visit.

Report, June 22nd : no attacks since middle of May, one week previous to first visit. Afraid of feeling better, as it meant in the past that an attack was due. Stamping and fidgeting of feet, a very prominent symptom in the past, much improved. I had thought of *Zinc.* for this symptom, but as he felt better it was thought best to leave well alone and continue with *Lycopodium.* Creasing of forehead, another *Lycopodium* symptom, well marked today; this creasing helps to relieve the pressure over the eyes : B.P. 125-70—urine dark red colour since being treated. R. *Lyc.* 12 nightly.

July 27th. No fit for nine weeks : is better than he has been for eighteen months : feeling of apprehension of legs giving way much less frequent; the feeling of expansion of head and balloon-like sensation much improved. Still has feeling of pitching forward; face not so pimply and less greasy. Continue non-meat diet; continue *Lyc.* 12.

September 7th. Eyes do not look so dark and shadowy and are

of a much deeper blue tint; gained over 2 pounds since June visit; has much more self-confidence; can pass places where he used to have attacks without fear; not so restless. No attacks for fifteen weeks. *Lyc.* 30.

October 19th. Lessening of all symptoms. Sleeps heavily, has giddy feeling from 5 to 8 a.m. which wears off after a few hours. No attack for twenty-one weeks: "feels as if he could take up all his old pursuits again." Continue treatment as before.

November 30th. Had mild "unconscious turn" one morning after an upset, and very long and heavy work the previous day; rested for half an hour and felt well for the next two days; feels very well now. Weight now almost 11 stone. Sleeping well. *Lyc.* 30 three doses.

January 25th, 1936. No attack for 5½ months except the "slight turn of unconsciousness" he had early in November; feels and looks much better. *Lyc.* 12 nightly.

March 28th, 1936. Much better; no medicine for five or six weeks; no epileptic fits. *Lyc.* 12 night and morning.

June 6th, 1936. Felt very quarrelsome four weeks ago. Felt as if he could quarrel with a stone. Nose bleeding while washing his face one day which relieved sensation of enlargement of heart; still on vegetarian diet; occasionally has fish for his mid-day meal. *Lyc.* 10*m.*

Last report by letter on October 26th "that he is quite well and free from attacks of any kind".

This young man had treatment for just over a year; was kept steadily under the influence of his constitutional remedy which was *Lycopodium* in different potencies, and the result was very gratifying, as there was no return of major epileptic fits for a period of eighteen months.

From the moment he was put on his remedy, a general improvement in his health, gain in weight, and improvement in his psychological make-up was perceptible: what more could you wish for? Life should be pleasant once more for this young man, still standing on the threshold of his life, and now minus the fear of being bowled over without warning by an epileptic fit. Homœopathy can—and does—cure epilepsy and would keep many young people out of the mental homes, if they were treated early enough, according to the law of Simillimum.

I am not claiming that *Lycopodium* is the cure for epilepsy;

it was *the* cure for this patient; another remedy might be required to produce like satisfactory results in regard to other epileptics. In every case the individual "make-up" must determine the individual cure.

THE CURE OF RARE SKIN DISEASE

Mrs. R., on waking up from the anæsthetic after the birth of her sixth child found that her infant aroused unusual interest among the members of the hospital staff. It was examined and re-examined, X-rayed and so forth, shown to all the medical visitors, until she got very much alarmed. Being her sixth infant, she suffered under no illusions that it was just kindly interest in a particularly handsome baby, she thought there must be something seriously the matter. She got no satisfaction, but, like the importunate widow, she persevered, until one of the specialists, annoyed with her insistence, brutally told her the truth, or what he considered the truth, that her baby had got a certain disease, rare but very fatal, that it meant it would not live more than six months. She was to keep it in the hospital, until the time of its demise.

Mother-like she was most indignant about this, and sought another opinion. She was more lucky than she knew, for she struck a Homœopath who cared not a hoot for specialists and their opinions, but only delved in the despised books of old masters, men greater than the present generation of bacteriologists, and other ologists who are lost in a welter of names, a maze of their own making, diagnosis-mad they are, and what is diagnosis after all but giving a pain or discolouration a name, the more outlandish the better; and a specialist is a person who does research work in a special variety of disease, and who can invent a few new names and put new tags to old troubles.

N.B.—One heard this illuminating story the other day: a doctor told a friend of mine that he was sending all his cases of polio-myelitis (infantile paralysis) to a certain man, he had done a great deal of research with regard to that disease. The friend asked pertinently: "Does he cure this polio-myelitis?" "Oh, no," was the answer, "it can't be cured."

Well, the indignant mother showed the stricken baby to this disciple of Hahnemann, who did not know the wonderful and fearful name of this rare and extraordinary disease, but what she did know was how to cure this medical puzzle.

The baby did present a weird picture. The infant was a deep purple-blue all over its spine. This purple extended right over the shoulders and right down the buttocks on to the thighs. The patch was as hard as a brick. You could make no impression on this hard, solid substance, and the mother told how rapidly it had been spreading since its birth, three weeks ago. In quite a short time the ugly deformity of the skin would have crept all over the body, and the poor thing would have died of this, as she would not have been able to breathe through the skin, a very important function which is essential to life.

The doctor remembered reading the description of a fatal case of a snake bite, the *Lachesis* poison, and it corresponded in appearance to this rare skin disease. So, very confidently, she told the harassed mother that something could be done for the little mite, and gave a dose of *Lachesis* 10*m*. There was no anxiety in the doctor's mind. The homœopathic law could not be wrong, and a cure was predicted.

The next week the child was seen again—a definite improvement. The disease had been stayed. In three weeks there was no purple discolouration anywhere. In five weeks you would not have known that there was anything amiss with the child. It had grown wonderfully. The mother, a rather stout, elderly party, was not able to feed her herself. So she was put on cow's milk and water and throve. She is now six months, weighs 16 pounds and is teething, as she should.

The mother is, woman-like, waiting until the child is over six months old, and then she intends to show the doctor the live baby. He will probably say that his diagnosis was wrong, but not that this particular disease could be cured. The name of this disease is *Sclerema Neo-natorum*, which translated means hardness of part of the skin of babies. Would not the original doctor make a fuss, if he had managed to cure this incurable disease! And all that was needed was one dose of snake poison.

There was no necessity to repeat the dose as the child was well. Isn't Homœopathy great, if it can do things like this? Just think if instead of a poor child out of a back street of London, it had been the heir of an old well-known family. And this is not an isolated example of the power of this despised Homœopathy, but it is repeated again and again all over the world, wherever there are followers of this science.

A professor of medicine declared the other day that Homœopathy had done nothing for medicine except that one Homœopath had invented an instrument for measuring the pulse-rate. I say to that professor : you have forgotten the first duty of a doctor is to heal people of their ailments and afflictions. Homœopathy does this in the majority of the cases every day and all day, and those unfortunate individuals who are past curing, they are relieved of their pain without turning them into drugmaniacs, cocaine-fiends, and other horrors. They are given mild, sleep-producing remedies, which do not lead to suicide, accidental or otherwise. This is not so spectacular as operations and examinations with elaborate instruments, but more comfortable and less harassing to the patient. Homœopathy is a branch of medicine, albeit an important one; it sets out to teach the science of healing according to definite laws.

Mind you, in theory it is most important to find out where the particular lesion is situated; and it is fascinating to look down a gastroscope and see the ulcers inside a stomach; or through a cystoscope and see the ulcers or stones inside a bladder; and it is most helpful to find the foreign body inside the bronchioles of a lung and hook it out through the bronchoscope. It would be impossible to find an impacted tooth, or a safety-pin in the lung without a bronchoscope; but the use of these scientific instruments should be limited to searching for foreign bodies, etc. One's point is "give honour where honour is due"—but do not unnecessarily subject a patient to the torture of passing such an instrument as a gastroscope or cystoscope just to satisfy scientific curiosity, and leave him without any treatment to ease his suffering, as happens so often.

This child whose early medical history is described, was alive two years afterwards; there was no sign of any pigmentation, no hardness of the skin. Unfortunately the parents moved out of the district, and it was lost sight of. Anyway, according to the textbooks, it could not survive six months after birth, Homœopathy proved this prophecy to be wrong.

CURE OF A BACKWARD CHILD

THE door of my consulting room opened gently, and on lifting my head I saw a gun pointing at me. I ducked my head and— no, it was not somebody after my hard-earned shekels, I saw the grinning face of a mischievous little imp of a boy friend of mine peering above the toy gun. I fully entered into the game and pretended to be alarmed, while he made the pretence of firing at me the whole time his mother was talking to me. What a difference in this boy of four, I thought, in the last six months! Then he would hide his face and not look at either friend or foe, a doctor was anathema to him, not a word could be got out of him, certainly I should never have expected him to ask me to play with him.

His medical history is very interesting. About eighteen months ago his mother brought him just after an attack of some childish infectious disease which confined him in a fever hospital for six months. I fancy it was diphtheria followed by scarlet fever, or the other way about, no matter. Anyway her own general practitioner had alarmed her by enumerating all the evil complications he might have as the result of all this, heart and kidney disease, and goodness knows what else!

Father was not best pleased about trusting his one and only precious son to the mercy of a mere woman. Mother prevailed, however, and father now sings quite a different song.

I found some unresolved pneumonia, right-sided, and the boy was very disagreeable, would not be examined even, cough worse in the early morning between 3 and 5 o'clock. *Kali carbonicum* 30 was given to the child, and some unmedicated tablets to keep father quiet. Next week saw a great improvement in the physical condition of the boy. He had a repeat of the *Kali carbonicum* two or three weeks later, and began to improve visibly, he put on weight, his weight at that time was less than it had been a year before. By the by, I forgot to mention that he had already attended a well-known children's specialist for six months the previous summer and had received his pet brand of emulsion—gallons of it—without the slightest effect on his weight or his nerves.

He was 26 pounds in October 1933, and gained 8 pounds in the following six months, not bad for a child who had refused to gain anything on malt and cod liver oil emulsion.

But there was no improvement in his nervous condition. He would not look at strangers, would not play with other children, a most irritating child to deal with. Psycho-analysis was suggested by somebody, I think. Probably he would have landed in a child guidance clinic later on. Suddenly on seeing the child after a little interval it flashed across my mind, of course, he has a *Baryta carbonica* nature. There was the timidity, the hiding, the fear of strangers. So he was promptly put on a course of *Baryta carbonica* 6 night and morning for some weeks. That was about four months ago; then an interval of weeks on nothing, and then a dose of *Baryta carbonica* 1m. one month ago. No further medicine has been required since, he has gained another 3 pounds, his mentality is that of a normal boy of four, full of fun and mischief, and everybody is pleased.

That is what Homœopathy does in a backward child, and this is not an isolated instance.

He is now four and weighs nearly 38 pounds, which is excellent for a child of his age, and the difference in his mentality!

P.S.—This happened three years ago; one has not seen this lad for many months; but his mother tells me he ails nothing, and that he gets on well at school and makes many friends. There is no complaint of any shyness or backwardness, rather the opposite!

A HOMŒOPATHIC JOKE

JANE, the first child of her young parents, was very ill. Everybody in the house was upset. Mother had not had her clothes off for nights, father telephoned several times a day to know how she was. The doctor was perturbed, as the distressing vomiting still went on, in spite of all the various medicines that were tried. The Great Man was called in to give weight to the doctor's opinion, but he was puzzled and talked learnedly of a germ that might have attacked the child. All he could suggest was another consultation on the following day and removal to the Children's Hospital for further investigation.

A friend of the family who had experienced the wonderful results of Homœopathy, heard of this illness, and discussed it with a doctor of the new school, who, on hearing the symptoms, "intense craving for cold water with vomiting almost as soon as it had been swallowed", suggested *Phosphorus* as the indicated remedy. But the parents were blind, and certainly would never hear of any unorthodox treatment.

But Miss A. was determined to give Homœopathy a chance. She found, on arriving at the house, how done-up the mother was, and how much she wanted recreation. So she sent her out for an hour's walk, and promised to look after Jane meanwhile. Poor Jane did look ill! She was lying back in her little cot, all white and death-like, and appeared barely conscious, and so weak after all that vomiting. For days she had not been able to keep anything down. Miss A. hesitated. Should she, or should she not, give the *Phosphorus* she had brought with her? The desire to help the child conquered, and the *Phosphorus* was secretly given, before the mother returned home.

The next day Miss A. rang up in fear and trembling, and enquired how dear little Jane was, to be told joyfully by the mother that the darling had quite suddenly taken a turn for the better. In fact when the two doctors had arrived, she had been playing very gaily with her toys in her pen and had crowed and laughed at them, and previously to that she had demanded and

eaten her usual breakfast and kept it down! The Great Man
was very astonished at this unexpected sequel, and talked
learnedly of "a food pocket in the stomach" that had suddenly
emptied itself, and after emptying allowed the rest of the food
to be retained. He had to say something—poor man—to cover
up his ignorance. The friend, who had secretly performed the
miracle by giving the *Phosphorus*, chuckled quietly to herself,
and shared the joke later with the Homœopath—this joke
against the old school prejudice.

You will want to know what happened to little Jane? Well,
she never looked back after this, and had no return of the
vomiting, and soon got fit and well again.

As one swallow does not make the summer, you will say,
neither does one case prove that this sudden recovery was due to
the *Phosphorus*. It was probably only a coincidence. But if you
watch and have much to do with sick folk, you will frequently
come across cases of gastritis who show these peculiarities—great
thirst, desire for cold water, constant nausea except when something cold is taken into the stomach, bringing up everything,
even the cold water for which there is such a craving, and which
comes back, as soon as it gets warm in the stomach. Give *Phosphorus* in a case like that, and you will cure the sickness very
rapidly. You get such a combination of symptoms in the vomiting
of early pregnancy, and the young mother will be very grateful
to you, if you relieve her of this unpleasant trouble so easily and
so quickly with *Phosphorus*. The accompanying symptom in a
pregnant woman is often : aversion to tea. This clinches it. *Phos.*
will cure.

Many years ago I had a serious case of protracted vomiting in
a young baby, when I was acting locum for another doctor in a
babies' ward. Nothing would help. So in desperation I sent round
some *Phosphorus*, and lo and behold! it did the trick at once.
Weeks later the other doctor rang me up and enquired what the
pills were which I had left in the ward, and which the nurses
had found so wonderfully efficacious in cases of gastritis. She was
rather incredulous, when I told her it was *Phosphorus*, as she had
never heard of it before. Being fairly broad-minded, she continued to give it, because she could not help noticing the
difference in the babies afterwards.

There are many other medicines for vomiting, and you will
not cure *all* cases of vomiting with *Phosphorus*; only those cases

which have this craving for cold water, this special great thirst for quantities of cold water, which eases the nausea at first and then is all pumped up again in a short time. And grown-ups will tell you that they have an aversion and great dislike for tea, even though they are very fond of it as a rule.

This attention to even the smallest detail is most important, if you wish to be able to cure people of their ills according to homœopathic rule.

RHEUMATISM

"RHEUMATISM is incurable!" exclaimed a learned Judge the other day. One wonders what bitter experiences lay behind this sweeping statement of the legal authority. Was he so far wrong, after all?

Shall we examine this conclusion in the light of modern medicine? Rheumatism is a common complaint and is caused by exposure to the elements, rain, wet overhead and underfoot, wind and cold. Men and women following outdoor occupations are frequent sufferers of rheumatism in its various manifestations. Policemen on point duty, lorry drivers, agricultural labourers, workmen in the building trade, charwomen, are all equally liable. Age makes very little difference, sex is no bar. The insurance societies state that annually many thousand work-hours are lost, many thousands of workmen are crippled and laid aside for weeks, and much money is paid out in sick pay, and industry loses time and money from this painful, though not necessarily fatal disease. What has the medical profession done about it?

Latterly much money has been spent in research, whatever that may mean; rheumatism clinics have been opened in various parts of the country; various spas have improved the facilities they provide for treatment. Expensive electrical apparatus has been installed in these clinics, thousands of pounds have been invested in the latest ultra-violet ray lamps; most of them will be out of date and old-fashioned in a year or two. Mercury vapour lamps and radiant heat lamps were all the rage some time ago; now it must be infra-red lamps, which are said to charm away all pain. Even this in some quarters is *ultra vires*; some other lamps with even shorter rays act more magically— that is : in the imagination of the electrical manufacturers. There is a section of the medical profession who frankly say they know nothing about these lamps and rather doubt their efficacy; they would pin their faith to foam baths. Some of the insurance companies are sending their crippled pensioners to the British spas, such as Bath and other places. There is a multitude of advice.

"You pays your money, and you takes your choice." There is, of course, still the old conservative type of doctor who swears by heroic doses of salicyclic acid and aspirin; others prefer the latest product of the large French or British drug-houses, which has to be inoculated or injected into the poor unfortunate victim, with sometimes dire results. One remembers one lady who after an injection of a highly vaunted product of a German firm which was given for rheumatism of the neck, found herself unexpectedly in the casualty ward of a General Hospital, and was then told she had suddenly fainted in a public vehicle and, as nobody could bring her round, she had been taken to the hospital and had lain there for hours. Proper knock-out drops, were they not? And after this ignominious exhibition of herself, was she any better? No, she felt much more ill than she had done before, and had to stay in bed for days and was so shaken by her unpleasant experience, that she could not travel in buses or trams without being seized with violent tremors. As ordinarily she was a very strong-minded, active person she did not like this state of affairs at all; she had bottles of strong tonic from the doctor which had made no difference at all to her state, nor to the original rheumatism. And do you know what set her right in a day or two, that she could ride in public vehicles, that she could move her neck without excruciating pain? Just a few doses of *Lachesis*: the homœopathic preparation of the South American rattlesnake. It was given to her: as her headaches were *Lachesis* headaches, she had the *Lachesis* heats, her pains were left-sided, and so on; her whole condition cried out for *Lachesis*; and, when she got it, everything cleared up, even the swelling of the neck muscles disappeared.

What about it, My Lord: is rheumatism curable? This lady, at any rate, can testify to it, that hers went quickly and without leaving any aftermath. Can Homœopathy produce any other witnesses? This positive case may only have been a fluke, a happy coincidence, and, being a member of a very exact and meticulous profession, he will require more evidence, before he will change his sentence. But we Homœopaths can produce many positive proofs of cures of rheumatism; our literature is full of such cures and, if living witnesses are wanted, they can be produced at will.

I recall the case of a sturdy six foot detective inspector, who had the classical signs of acute rheumatic fever: swollen joints, acute pains, sour sweats, high temperatures; he was booked for

at least six weeks in bed, if not more. His temperature came
down in three days, his sweats ceased in less than a week, and he
was up and about in a little over three weeks, minus a weak
heart, and as strong and hefty as before, and he never had even
a grain of salicyclic acid or a single pill of aspirin! Nor was he
rubbed with liniment. He was given metallic *Mercury* in minute
doses; in old-school medicine Mercury is reserved for syphilitic
cases, but there was no syphilis in this inspector's past history;
and yet his symptoms were pathognomonic of *Mercury*, at least
to a follower of Hahnemann; and, strangely enough, *Mercury*
cured rapidly and so quickly that the police surgeon who had to
pay weekly visits in order to make official reports to the authorities, was astonished himself. The symptoms pointing to *Mercury*
were as follows: very offensive sweats, the more the patient
sweated, the worse he felt, he was so exhausted and so weary, he
was only comfortable in bed, and yet as soon as he got warm in
bed, he had to throw off his bedclothes, then he felt cold and
his pains got worse again and he covered himself again, and so
it went on the whole time. He hated the nights: all his pains, all
his discomfort were worse during the night. His tongue was
thickly furred; he presented the picture of a man who had taken
an overdose of Mercury, a common enough sight in the venereal
wards in the old days. And as I said before, *Mercury* in small
doses acted rapidly and cured him.

Acute rheumatic fever takes anything from six to fourteen
weeks or more to recover from as a rule; past experience in the
wards of the large teaching hospitals has taught one, that this
is so. And there seems to be very little change in the results
obtained nowadays with the latest treatment. Patients still report
a stay of many weeks in hospital, if rheumatic fever is diagnosed;
and to find later that homœopathic treatment shortens the course
of a wearisome and expensive disease, such as rheumatic fever, is
most gratifying. I may be allowed at this point to stress the
importance of the financial costs of a lengthy illness: it affects
industry, as it may be a valuable worker who is laid low; it
affects the insurance societies who have to pay out more money;
and it affects the individual worker and his family, as, when a
man is losing his income, the family has to live on the savings, if
any, or miserably subsist on the small sick pay. And it also affects
the ratepayer's pocket, as a bed is being occupied for weeks by
one person at a considerable cost. If the time of stay could be

reduced, there would be an all-round gain. If the medical profession and the hospitals would only realize what has been done for acute diseases under homœopathic treatment, the lot of the individual patient would be much happier.

I shall be told that I have not proved my case by just quoting one patient's history. I shall therefore mention another case; she was a middle-aged woman, the mother of a large family. She had rheumatic fever, but the minute details of her illness were very different from the case I mentioned previously: there was practically no perspiration, she was not very restless, as movement definitely made the pains worse, warmth relieved the acute pains, the warm bed, the warm flannel dressing relieved, the pains were wandering, shifting ones, that is one day one joint was affected, the next day a totally different joint was more swollen and inflamed, one day she had diarrhœa and that day her pains hardly troubled her. I did not spot the remedy straight away, but after a few days it became clear to me that *Kali bichrom.* was the correct medicine, and after that we had very little trouble; I remember the nurse was horrified, because I would not allow any oil of winter green to be used, or any friction with turpentine liniment. In the end she expressed her surprise that the case had turned out to be such a mild one, it had got well so quickly. I cannot recall the length of time this lady was ill; the temperature came down in less than a week and she was, I fancy, up and about in well under the six weeks.

These two were both severe cases in the beginning, and had taken a good hold of the respective people, before they came under medical care, and were on that account all the greater credit to homœopathic treatment.

Now we shall leave the subject of acute rheumatic fever and tackle the more common and more widely spread muscular rheumatism.

There are very few people in our damp Northern atmosphere who have not at some time or other experienced the agonizing pains of acute lumbago. The attack lasts, under ordinary treatment with aspirin and liniment, about ten to fourteen days; outwardly there is very little to show to account for the crippling effect lumbago has on its victims, and yet there you are, chained to your bed, and even the King's horses and the King's men could not drag you forth again without shrieks of agony, in spite of mocking laughter. And what can Homœopathy do for you in such humiliating circumstances? It can be the fairy who, with her magic wand, releases you from your prison, so that you are able to join in the midnight dance and revels of hobgoblins, should you so desire. This is not an exaggeration nor a figure of speech, but hard fact. Listen to this: A young office worker had to travel on top of an open bus on a teeming morning; she got well drenched and could not shed her wet garments until the evening, with the result that the next morning she was fixed in bed with a full-blown attack of lumbago. The following details were elicited: pain on first beginning to move and easier after continued motion, restlessness which compelled her to move all the time, this combined with the cause of the attack, namely the rain and the wetting, pointed to *Rhus. tox.*, and *Rhus tox.* cleared up this annoying complaint so that she could get back to work within twenty-four hours. This is not an isolated case, but I have repeated this rapid cure again and again with the same remedy.

Sometimes *Bryonia* is required in alternation with *Rhus tox.* In a *Bryonia* case you would find the *Bryonia* characteristics most outstanding, such as: the pain comes on as soon as he moves, and any movement is so excruciating that he has to lie absolutely still; coughing and sneezing is agonizing, but firm pressure is soothing and grateful. Wherever you find rheumatism whether in the back muscles or in the neck or in the limbs, provided these details are present, *Bryonia* will cure. I remember a case in a young woman where *Bryonia* and *Rhus tox.* were tried with very little benefit; then it was noticed that the patient was rather tearful, that she had to move, kept on moving to get any ease; here *Puls.* was prescribed, and within less than twenty-four hours, this young woman was out of her bed and anxious to return to her job. *Bry., Puls.* and *Rhus tox.* are very much alike; but one remedy will not do for another. For the best and quickest results get to know the characteristics of each one.

After two years of drought, England is once more living up to its reputation of grey, weeping skies and damp muddy roads, and we shall get again our usual crop of rheumatism and allied diseases due to exposure to wet, though there is another class of case which is more affected by heat and dry atmosphere. I recall the pathetic wail of a man in one of the daily papers in which he condemns the incompetence of the medical profession for being

unable to deal successfully with such common or garden complaints as rheumatism, and "can somebody tell me," he plain-
tively writes, "why rheumatism, which is a wet weather disease,
comes on with me during the height of summer. If it is a brilliantly warm cloudless day, I am crippled, and, moreover, when
I get into bed and get comfortable and hot, then my enemy,
rheumatism, begins to plague me, and doctors only shrug their
shoulders and do nothing." One wished that this poor man could
have been introduced to Homœopathy. He describes the pains
which are found under *Sulphur*, and which *Sulphur* alone would
rapidly remove. A *Sulphur* patient revels in damp and cold, he
is limber and active in the damp, but during a dry, warm, sum-
mery spell, he gets the knees of a worn-out cabhorse, painfully
and stiffly he drags along. He hates the nights, for the warmth of
the bed heats up his muscles so that they burn and ache, and he
has to search for the cool places in the bed or hang his feet out,
and how easily he gets cured, once he gets under the right
régime! It may be just muscular rheumatism or myalgia or
rheumatic fever, or even that dreaded rheumatoid arthritis,
where the deeper structures of the joints are affected. If you find
these symptoms, *Sulphur* will help : quickly in muscular rheumatism and more slowly in rheumatic fever; you have to repeat
the doses more often in an acute inflammatory condition, and
where there are organic changes, such as you find in arthritis,
you will have to wait some time, before the recuperative forces of
nature are able to undo the damage that has been done and
loosen up the stiffened joints.

There was a lady who came some time ago from the West of
England with the tag "Arthritis." She had been crippled with
arthritis of the left knee for over a year or more, and was unable
to do much or enjoy life with her husband. Her sister had been
cured very quickly by Homœopathy some years previously of
her rheumatic knee by alternative doses of *Rhus. tox.* and
Bryonia; a very favourite prescription of mine, *if* the symptoms
agree, and one has the authority of Hahnemann for this alternation. Well, this good lady arrived, her left knee was stiff, she
could not bend it at all and had to sit very gingerly on the edge
of the chair with her leg out in front of her. There was tighten-
ing of the hamstring muscles at the back of the knee, but no
definite involvement of the knee joint; she could not kneel, and
walking was a great trial to her. The symptoms again worked

out to *Rhus. tox.* and *Rhus. tox.* 6 in pellets, three times daily, was prescribed. I did not see her again for six months or so. For some reason or another she had been unable to come up to town to report, but had continued with the pellets, and when she paid the second visit, she was able to bend the knee, and there was only a slight tenseness of the muscles behind the knee, and then at the third visit she only came to report complete recovery : she was as spry as ever she had been before, and marvelled only how a few small pellets could make such a difference, when all the other remedies she had tried, had proved a failure. Yes, *Rhus. tox.* is a miracle worker in rheumatic troubles, if you have *Rhus. tox.* symptoms, the exposure to damp, the stiffness and pain on first beginning to move, which will disappear on continued motion.

There is fibrositis, a new favourite diagnosis of the present-day Æsculapius, which is only another name for the old-fashioned rheumatism. You feel the hard nodules in the muscles which are so painful to touch and movement, and which take such ages to remove with massage and hot air baths and radiant heat, etc. By the by, don't put a *Sulphur* patient into hot air baths or give him radiant heat, and if by chance he is a peppery old colonel, you will hear about it, if you start up his pains with the radiant heat or the infra red rays. Give the patient with the fibrotic nodules the remedy which is indicated by his symptoms, and if they are only recent nodules, they will melt away in a very short time; if they are old and thick, they will take longer, but they will go, too. I am not decrying such auxiliary measures as infra red lamps or Turkish baths or radiant heat. They are very soothing and comforting and often very helpful, and sometimes when the indicated homœopathic medicine takes a long time to act, which in a long-standing chronic case is often the case, all these necessary accessory measures are of use, as the individual patient feels something is being done, and the psychological effect of coloured lamps and infra red rays is not to be despised.

I remember a case far advanced with rheumatoid arthritis, there were the typical pear-shaped swellings of the wrists and ankles : she was not able to raise her arms in order to attend to her hair even; she was brought at first in a bath chair, as she could not walk. I don't know how many years she had been like it. She had radiant heat and infra red heat; faithfully she came twice a week for two years, and gradually the distorted joints took on a more normal appearance, the movements became freer and easier. She could do her own hair, she discarded her bath chair and came tripping along on her own feet. She was able to discard various artificial appliances to correct flat foot, and she was very pleased with herself. But I was not; the moment she gave up her light treatment, back would come the pains, and the muscles would tighten up again. I bethought myself, why not try homœopathic medication? I know some of the homœo-pathic writers do not hold out much hope in advanced cases of crippling arthritis, but why not try? I took some of the symp-toms, and I found that she was a gentle, timid soul, easily moved to tears, affected by warm weather, even though she liked warmth for her local aches and pains; she disliked fat food, and *Pulsatilla* was so plainly her constitutional remedy that she was given *Pulsatilla*. And after three months on *Pulsatilla* continuous with artificial sunlight treatment, the progress was not only more rapid, but it was maintained without the aid of further light baths. This is over two years ago. Nobody would know nowadays, looking at her joints, that she had arthritis, she has had no return of pain or crippling stiffness and deformity, and has had no treatment during all this time. And she continues well, so the report goes. The remarkable point was that three months' homœopathic treatment equalled in her case nearly one year's treatment without it. That is : her progress during the last three months under Homœopathy was very much quicker than during the twelve months on light treatment alone, and, more-over, it was maintained. A very satisfactory result from the patient's point of view.

Some time ago it was mentioned in the Press that bee-keepers very rarely suffered from rheumatism, and the bright suggestion was made that people should allow themselves to be stung in order to cure their rheumatism. A very painful and unpleasant procedure! The homœopaths have known of the action of the bee poison in rheumatism for over 100 years, ever since Hahne-mann's days in the eighteenth century. But it only acts in a certain type of rheumatism, and only through the homœopathic way of taking a case and finding the symptoms can you cure the kind of rheumatism which yields to *Apis*, the poison of the honey bee, and you do not often come across *Apis* symptoms, except in acute inflammation of the joints. I remember the case of a nurse who presented such an *Apis* picture : inflammation of the right knee joint which looked red, felt hot to touch and pitted on pressure. There was œdema all round; she complained of stinging and burning pains in the joints which were worse in the warm bed, worse hot application, worse sitting near the warm stove: all this nearly drove her crazy. I found her sitting up in a cold room with the knee exposed to the cold air, and a basin of cold water near her, which she applied to her knee to cool the burning and stinging in the joints. I soon saw that this could only be *Apis,* and *Apis* 1*m*, four-hourly, was prescribed, and the relief was instantaneous almost. In twenty-four hours the swelling had gone down, and a week later the patient was back at work.

It is no use applying the bee poison to all and sundry rheumatic patients, you would have many failures; it would only do good in those cases which present the typical *Apis* symptoms: the swelling, œdema, redness, tenderness to touch, the burning, stinging pains which are made worse by heat. Take each case of rheumatism individually, and find out the particulars, the aggravations, the ameliorations of the pains, the cause of the rheumatism, and you will get cures in almost every case.

I remember a young woman, she had been to the winter sports and came back crippled with rheumatism. I found out that she had become hot skating, it was brilliant sunshine, she had thrown off some of her clothes, suddenly a cold wind had come up, the sun had gone behind clouds, and it had begun to snow. The result of the sudden change from hot to a cold temperature and the exposure to cold, damp snow plus the suppressed perspiration, had led to rheumatism of the neck muscles and back. This was a typical *Dulcamara* case, and *Dulcamara* speedily put her right. You will get *Dulcamara* rheumatism frequently in climates where there are great differences in temperature within twenty-four hours, and which in England occurs more in the autumn, when warm sunny days are followed by cold nights, especially if there is a cold damp atmosphere, and if heavy rain follows on a warm day.

I remember another patient, she was an elderly woman who suffered a great deal from stiffness in the neck and pains in the head, shooting, tearing pains, so that she had to wrap up her neck and head to get relief. These pains were always worse in cold wet weather. I tried *Dulcamara* with very little benefit. On further enquiry she volunteered the information that she always

knew when there was thunder about, for the pains became unbearable before a thunder storm. *Rhododendron* has such an
aggravation before thunder storms, and *Rhod.* 1*m.*, four-hourly,
for a week, cleared up the pains and the stiffness which had
lasted for many weeks.

"*Stiff neck*" is quite a common rheumatic affection : *Rhus.
tox.* and *Bryonia* often help, but there is another remedy which
has a particular relationship to the muscles of the nape of the
neck, and that is the American plant, *Cimicifuga* : a Black
Cohosh. Shall we quote a case illustrating the effect this medicine
has ? A stout middle-aged woman was seen at the Dispensary :
her head was drawn back, and she could not turn it either to the
right or the left. She could not lie on her back, because the muscles
of the back were tightly contracted, neither could she lie on her
side, because the muscles jumped and jerked. She was extremely
depressed and gloomy about her condition, nothing could do her
any good, she could not get well, she was done. It was no use
trying. She was persuaded to try the *Cimicifuga*; she was not
told, of course, what she had. She thought she got some kind of
aspirin; but it was *Cimicifuga* in a very minute dosage—in fact
Cimicifuga 30, three-hourly, and the next time she was seen all
the depression and gloom had gone; the muscles of the nape of
the neck were soft and flexible. She could turn her head, whichever way she wished, and all this in less than forty-eight hours.
And for a wonder she was quite grateful! The late Dr. Clarke
speaks very highly of the action of the resinoid *Macrotin* found
in this plant. He usually used the *Macrotin* in the 3*x* trituration
for lumbago and stiff neck. One has not so far had occasion to
use this resinoid, but should a case come along with the *Cimicifuga* particulars, and which does not respond to the higher
potencies, one would then apply the *Macrotin* on Dr. Clarke's
authority and expect a cure.*

A variety of remedies have been mentioned which cure different forms of rheumatism; but there are many more medicines
which cure this disease homœopathically. Their number, indeed, is very extensive : Kent's *Repertory* gives 118 different
names under the rubric "Rheumatism"; so you see homœopathic

* *Macrotin* 3*x*. 2 doses in 12 hours, completely cured for me a case
of right-sided sciatica of several weeks' standing, without any subsequent
return of the agonising pains.

doctors are well supplied with drugs which can and do cure this painful disease under its various manifestations.

Ask an allopathic doctor, what is his stand-by in rheumatism or rheumatic fever or even rheumatoid arthritis, he will tell you without hesitating a moment that Salicylic acid or one of its salts are absolutely specific: they are Salicylate of Soda, Salicine, aspirin which is Acetyl-Salicylic acid—Salol or Phenol, Salicylate—all are used more or less without discrimination. Some favour one medicine, some another. Salicylic acid is found in the bark and leaves of willows; and it only became known round about 1876 in Europe that South African natives used infusion of willow-tips for clearing up rheumatic disorders. Medical science does not like infusions, but prefers to extract what is called the active principles, which are too concentrated in their actions and too violent. One cannot deny that the salicylates frequently remove the pains, but as such enormous doses are used, they are followed by all kinds of after results: dizziness, giddiness, delirium and gastric upsets and prostration. But the medico is pleased, the pains have gone and the patient is most times so weak he can't object; and then he is dosed up with noxious bitter tonics and it takes him weeks to get over the combined effects of the disease and the overdosing.

I remember one such tiresome case of rheumatic fever which occurred in the early days of my medical career, while acting as an assistant to a very good general practitioner. I *had to treat* the patients allopathically and this particular case gave me many anxious hours; even though I had the moral support of my chief and several specialists. This good lady developed acute rheumatic fever during the war as a result of exposure during a snowy wintry spell. She was a very headstrong, self-willed party and liked to order her own treatment, and thought she knew all about how to cure herself. She ruled the whole house from her bedside with an iron hand, maids, nurses, specialists, and poor me had no chance to stand up against her. The acute rheumatic fever was followed by pericarditis, endocarditis, double pleurisy with effusion; the temperature became swinging, going up to between 103° and 104° every night and dropping down to 99° every morning. So it went on, week after week, month after month; several times she nearly died, but still she hung on to life with a grim persistence.

In the end, after a nine months' illness, she was a pathetic sight, "sans teeth, sans hair," it had all fallen out; so weak she could not even raise a finger to fasten a button, she was nothing but a skeleton, the skin was just hanging loose over her bones, and there was an enormous collection of fluid in her abdomen, a tubercular peritonitis. I have often noticed since that tuberculosis is closely related to rheumatism; and tubercular families produce more cases of rheumatism than other families who are not tubercular. The specialists shrugged their shoulders, nothing more could be done. She had had all the different varieties of salicylates in small and ever-increasing dosages, and official medicine was stumped. She received the last rites of her faith and awaited the end, quite indomitable, even to the last.

She had no longer got sufficient strength to question the treatment she was receiving, so *Tuberculinum* 30, one dose, was given, the next day the temperature only went up to 101.8° instead of 104°; I was on the right track, I thought, at last. Then the *Repertory* was made use of and after much searching a remedy was found which corresponded to her symptoms, mind you, not her physiological or pathological state, no notice was taken of diagnosis, her rheumatic fever, her past rheumatic-tubercular condition, the tubercular peritonitis. But I only considered and looked up her little idiosyncrasies, the extreme weakness following prolonged fever, the great and excessive general emaciation, the withering of the limbs, the falling out of the hair, her inability to take lemonade and any stimulants such as wines and alcohol in any form, which was followed by diarrhœa; also diarrhœa after any fruit, diarrhœa after tea, so weak even after first waking up after a long sleep, extreme sensitiveness to the slightest draught even to a current of warm air. All this was found in the *Repertory* and pointed to *Selenium*. I had not got *Selenium*, I had not even heard of it before; but according to the tenets of the homœopathic laws, *Selenium* was indicated, and therefore a hurried visit was made to the chemist, and *Selen.* 30 was obtained as a last resource.

I hardly dared to hope for any results, the patient was really too far gone. The next day arrived; I almost hesitated to ring the bell; the nurse opened the door.

"Doctor, what was in that powder you gave her yesterday morning, the temperature went down to normal and remained normal during the last twenty-four hours, the first time for nine months?"

And from that moment everything changed with a dramatic suddenness, the temperature never went up again, the hectic flush disappeared from her face, the white smooth hairless scalp began to cover itself with hair again, the limbs filled out, the fluid in the abdomen became gradually less and less; the diarrhœa disappeared. The single dose of *Selenium* 30 remained active for eight weeks, then three more doses were given in quick succession, and no further medicine was required; no tonics—nothing. Three months after the first dose was given, she started to walk again and five months afterwards her weight was up again to 8 stones and she was discharged as cured and sent to the seaside. Ten years later she was still alive and active; no recurrence of her disease, heart and lungs and abdomen were sound.

That was the effect of a very few powders of the indicated homœopathic remedy—prescribed according to the law that like cures like—and such unexpected cures any good Homœopath who follows closely in the footsteps of the great master Hahnemann, can produce by the score.

These cures are not accidental, one can explain the reason. There is no need to boast. The same thing has been done ever since Hahnemann discovered the laws of Homœopathy, the books are full of such cures and they happen every day in the practices of the many thousands of homœopathic practitioners all over the world. These cures are not happy flukes, but hard facts.

A very similar case, though not so extreme, occurred during this last year. An elderly lady developed a mysterious illness after exposure to wet, and the temperature would not go down for weeks. She was sent into hospital and there all kinds of tests were made : blood tests, serum tests, bismuth meals, X-rays, etc., and no cause could be found for this mysterious pyrexia. There was no T.B., no cancer, but the temperature remained up for five months, and the patient became weaker and weaker, and emaciated more and more.

There was diarrhœa, pain after drinking tea, inability to take fruit, so once more *Selenium* 30 was prescribed, with the same happy effects; it had to be repeated more frequently and was then followed by *Sulphur*. The temperature dropped and the mysterious nameless disease cleared up. On closer enquiry I discovered she had had many rheumatic pains in the arms, shoulders and neck, for several months in the beginning; but nobody had paid much attention to this, so I can only presume that this was a kind of low rheumatic fever, which cleared up after the appropriate remedies.

Now we shall leave the acute type of rheumatic fever and go back to the more chronic kind of muscular rheumatism. I recall to mind an old age pensioner who brought her little grandchild to the dispensary for heart trouble. The old granny herself was very feeble and for two weeks she did not turn up, then she made another visit and arrived in a very pitiable condition. She came crawling along, holding on to chairs and tables, her body bent double like the letter Z; the pain was all in the sacrum and went into the hips and was agonizing when she walked, almost impossible for her to rise after sitting. I recognized the remedy, and the old lady received *Æsculus hippocastanum*—horse-chestnut in the 6th potency, four-hourly. The next week she came in full of smiles, her poor old back had straightened itself, she walked erect, pains and stiffness practically gone. Isn't it worth while to get results like this, and that in a lady nearly eighty years of age !

"Have I proved my case, My Lord? that rheumatism in its various forms is curable by Homœopathy"; and I have only mentioned a few cases, picked out at random.

Intricate law cases are argued before the judge in chambers; and the various counsels produce many tomes, many books to prove the various points that are raised; the Homœopaths also have many learned books, many learned authorities from whom they quote, who for nearly 200 years now have shown how to cure rheumatism and many other diseases. There is Professor Kent who has written many big books, there is old Dr. John Clarke who gives many examples in his writings of how to set about to cure rheumatism, and gives case after case of cures. There is Carrol Dunham, there is Professor Farringdon, there is Boenninghausen; there are American and German and French and British writers, old and long dead authorities, who still live in their books. There are men who are alive today and daily reproduce the same cures in rheumatism as the old masters : "My Lord, Homœopathy is alive, very much alive, and it can cure rheumatism," and it has cured it in the past, cures it now and will cure it in the future.

A CURE OF RHEUMATOID ARTHRITIS

At the beginning of January, a poor woman came to me about her little boy who was suffering from a minor complaint, the real patient was herself. She came hobbling in, almost bent double, leaning on two sticks.

"Hullo," I exclaimed, "what have you been doing to yourself?" "Oh," she answered, "I have got rheumatoid arthritis and the doctor at the hospital says I can't be cured, it can only be relieved with electrical treatment. As I have no time to sit and wait at hospital, I must just get on as best I can."

I persuaded her to let me have a look at the offending member. On uncovering the legs I found both knees very much swollen. It took three extensions of the hands to encircle each knee, they looked red and inflamed and stiff; in my opinion there was certainly serious trouble in both the joints. On the other hand, I did not agree with the prognosis, that is, with the conclusion the hospital specialist had drawn.

I asked a few apparently senseless questions, which yielded the following result : the trouble started five months ago in her right knee, it then attacked the left knee as well; she always felt much worse in the afternoon. She was of a yielding nature, rather timid; and I had enough to work upon. The veriest tyro in Homœopathy could guess the right remedy; so one dose of *Lycopodium* in the 30th potency was given to her and she was instructed to present herself again in a week's time. There was no attempt made to diet her. I was promising myself to go into that more fully at the next visit.

Several weeks passed; no Mrs. B. arrived! After six weeks she was seen accidentally by one of the staff, minus her two sticks. "Well, no need to ask you how you are," said the sister, "you look heaps better, and walking quite upright, too, without any support." "Oh," Mrs. B. replied, "I can walk all right, but I have still got some pain in the knees." She was then persuaded to present herself for a further examination, when I found her knees had almost returned to normal size; there was no redness, just a little stiffness, and some slight locking of the joint. She was then reassured that everything was going on as well as, and better than, I had expected and that, as a matter of fact, she was well on the road to recovery, and she was then given another dose of *Lycopodium* 30.

Poor thing, she was rather overwhelmed. "But the doctor at the hospital said I could never get better," she kept on repeating, "he could do nothing more for me!" So there she is, after only six weeks, walking upright without any artificial aid whatever, only a little pain, and some locking of the joints.

In a few more weeks this also should be gone. Of course, there was as yet no bony deformity, the arthritis being of comparatively recent origin, yet, let it be emphasized—she was supposed to be incurable!

Notwithstanding, within two days of starting the homœopathic treatment, she had thrown away her sticks, and could walk upright without extraneous assistance.

Surely this "gives one to think," and the student of homœopathic medicine will find it well worth while to study a system that will operate effectively, as in this case, without any effort on the patient's part, and with so little outward show.

HOMŒOPATHY IN FIRST AID

"ACCIDENTS will happen in the best regulated families," and however careful one is, falls and tumbles occur, and serious injuries may come to any one of us.

The value of homœopathic medication can be tried out by anyone who is wondering whether there is anything in the claim of this school that *"Like cures Like."*

The orthodox recommendation is: to apply iodine to the injured skin to prevent any bacterial infection; if there is serious injury and shock, morphia is given hypodermically to kill pain, and prevent and counteract shock. Now, Homœopathy presents you with a more pleasant alternative, and you do not need to wait for morphia; and even the iodine will not be required, for iodine may cause serious burns to sensitive skins, as has been seen again and again.

The homœopathic way is to apply *Arnica* locally in a weak, watery solution, and also to give it internally, by the mouth. If you are doubtful of its action, try it in the 3rd decimal and you will be agreeably surprised how quickly it relieves the pain in even serious injuries, and how it counters shock. Many patients thought they were being given morphia, when all they had was *Arnica* in some potency or other, which acted rapidly and beneficently, without leaving any drug action behind, or any craving for further doses of morphia. Many cases of morphia drug-addicts can be traced back to the first dose which a kindly doctor gave to soothe and palliate pain.

"Arnica," many sceptics have said—and *will* say—"is only an old wives' simple, and you might just as well apply cold water to the injured surface: it will do as much good; there is no medicinal action in *Arnica*; the relief is entirely due to the cold water!"

Leave the sceptics to their unbelief! I have known, and experienced and seen, in others and myself, the marvellous pain-killing effects of *Arnica* in injuries.

An old age pensioner, after having spent a long evening in the local public house with his cronies, staggered homewards at closing time, singing gaily and raucously at the top of his voice. Malignant fate overtook him; he quarrelled with the kerb and kissed the ground and was brought home unconscious with a gashed head. Whether the unconsciousness was due to the fumes of alcohol, or due to concussion, I could not decide, offhand, but knowing how quarrelsome the inebriated can be, I let well alone; cleaned up his head, found the extent of the damage, and put in four stitches without waking him. The son, an ambulance driver, was anxious to take the gay reprobate to the infirmary, in case there was more serious injury to the brain. Meanwhile, I gave a dose of *Arnica*, and while still discussing the advisability of fetching the ambulance with the family, the old gentleman stirred—it was less than five minutes after the dose—opened one eye, and enquired what had happened to him. The dose of *Arnica* had done what the washing, the stitching up and dressing his wound, and putting him to bed had failed to do—had wakened and roused him. As his pulse was stronger and more regular he was left in the bosom of his family and ordered *Arnica* in four-hourly doses.

By next morning a very chastened convalescent old man was ready to receive me; nothing further of importance occurred; in a few days the stitches were removed and his recovery was complete.

Now for some personal experiences.

While making a rockery a stone rolled off the home-made trolley and fell on, and crushed, one of my fingers. The agony was intense; cold sweat ran down my face; one felt, and looked, green—and I was never nearer fainting than on this occasion! Cold tap water was run on the hand, but the pain was as severe as before; then the hand was put in cold *Arnica* lotion, and *Arnica* 30 was taken. Within an incredibly short time relief set in; the cold sweat and the pain disappeared. I put on an *Arnica* dressing and took *Arnica* 30 four-hourly, and had no further anxiety or pain, though the nail turned black and blue and remained so for days, and I did not even lose the nail!

Another time I slipped and knocked my head against a stone wall. I saw stars, and was dazed for an appreciable time. Three-quarters of an hour elapsed before I reached home and by that time a beautiful, egg-shaped swelling with enlarged veins over it had come up on my temple, and there was an abrasion of the skin as well, and my head ached furiously! No iodine was applied locally; I only took some *Arnica*, internally, and with great interest watched the swelling on my forehead recede! Within an hour it had gone, and by next morning there was not even a bruise left. I was thankful to be spared the embarrassment of walking about with a blackened eye and forehead!

Arnica has justified its use in all kinds of accidents; fractures, dislocations and motor-car accidents, and it never lets one down; the relief is instantaneous. One word of warning, though; do not use pure *Arnica* locally. It causes an eruption of the skin, an unpleasant dermatitis, almost like erysipelas: use a diluted solution of *Arnica* for bruises, and if there is any skin abrasion, use a solution of the herb *Calendula* to dress the wound. It acts more pleasantly and safely than stronger antiseptics.

During the War, Dr. Petrie Hoyle, that keen fighter for recognition of the value of Homœopathy, used *Calendula* almost exclusively for dressing the most filthy wounds in his front-line hospital, and he was commended by a visiting Staff Officer for the clean state of the patients' wounds; the absence of smell in the wards, and received much praise on the rapid evacuation and cure of all kinds of septic wounds among the soldiers. They had no fatal cases of gas gangrene among the patients, I believe.

And all this was due to the action of the *Calendula* lotion, and the indicated homœopathic remedies, and no other antiseptics were used in suppurating wounds.

These cures are another proof of the validity of the law of "similars," even in surgery.

A friend of Hahnemann, a Dr. Franz, took repeated doses of tincture of *Calendula officinalis* (Marigold). These doses of *Calendula* so affected an old scar left by a wound that it became very raw and sore, and threatened to suppurate; he also began to shiver and developed a temperature. Therefore, Dr. Franz concluded that as *Calendula* evidently caused suppuration in wounds, if taken in large doses, it should, in small doses, cure suppuration in wounds!

Hence Dr. Hoyle's success, many years later, in the French War Hospital.

Indeed, I have used *Calendula* lotion when suturing a lacerated perineum in maternity cases, and I have not regretted it. I have never seen a cleaner wound surface or more rapid healing in a torn perineum than those which were treated with *Calendula* sprays, and it was much more efficacious, and more rapid,

than the strongest antiseptic, nor was there any rise in temperature after!

I should rely on *Calendula* and *Arnica* and *Hypericum* lotion
in treatment of injuries, and wounds and suppurations in preference to all the mercurial and carbolic lotions and other antiseptics of the orthodox!

Mr. Carleton, an American surgeon, who wrote an excellent,
practical work on *Homœopathy in Medicine and Surgery* is my
authority for the use of *Calendula* in obstetric and gynecological
practice. He used it freely in all his gynecological cases, and never
expected—and never had—any sepsis, following this treatment.
It is a relief to be able to use such mild lotions as *Calendula* and
Hypericum; they do not play such havoc with one's hands, as do
the mercurial lotions, or the various brands of lysol.

All first aid equipment should contain *Arnica* tincture, and
lotion, and *Hypericum* for external use; *Arnica* in pilule form
for shock and collapse; *Calendula* lotion, applied pure, stops
severe hæmorrhage very rapidly, as a veterinary nurse taught me,
who used it neat for applying to four days old puppies, after
docking their tails.

Antisepsis is overrated; use Asepsis, and strict cleanliness, and
the tinctures and lotions made from various herbs, and always
with the relative medicinal remedy, *Arnica*, and so forth; and so
prove beyond doubt, the soundness of the homœopathic principle
—"Like cures Like."

FIRST AID IN PRACTICE

As the years roll on and with greater experience, I am more convinced than ever of the importance of the prevention of disease, particularly in accidents and injuries. The period of incapacity can be shortened and unnecessary suffering can be avoided by the proper knowledge and application of the homœopathic remedies, not forgetting the well-tried aseptic herbal lotions, tinctures and ointments.

Some personal experiences will not come amiss here. Do not forget that for many years, although I used homœopathic medicines internally as well as externally in my private practice in my capacity of medical officer at a public health institution, I felt that the nursing staff would be too biassed to carry out my instructions if I strayed from the orthodox paths. I had learnt early in my professional life that sisters and nurses only carry out the directions of the visiting doctors which coincided with their own ideas, and unless a surgeon or a physician personally saw to it, half the instructions would not be carried out. Then this last war came along, and with it a change of staff. At first my work at the Dispensary was shattered, wiped out by the stroke of a pen.... The youngsters, almost over night were removed into so-called safe areas—safe on paper—thus breaking up the sanctity of the home and destroying all family ties, by scattering the various members of a family from the crowded cities, over the unwilling and reluctant countryside. Doctors, lawyers and other professional men found themselves without work at one go. A minimum of sane parents preferred to keep their children with them, defying the instructions of autocratic officialdom, preferring the threats of hypothetical bombs to separation from their loved ones. In due course the air raids materialised, only the German airmen did not have the politeness to enquire at Whitehall first, which were reception areas or safe areas in their opinion and which were danger zones; but scattered their dangerous missiles wherever they chose, on lonely country as well as on closely-populated cities. After a few months of interregnum of closure of schools, the Education authorities were forced to re-open some of them, as well as some of the health clinics, for the sake of the children left behind who were running wild in the streets. The staff at the clinic now consisted of one trained nurse and the caretaker. Both were exceedingly valuable, the sister proved herself a tower of strength, willing and only too anxious to carry out to the letter the orders given. For almost the first time I found willing co-operation. We scrapped the antiseptics; decided for a time to use nothing but herbal tinctures, lotions and ointments and to give homœopathic remedies a thorough trial. If the herbal lotions did not work better than the orthodox methods, we could always go back to the old ways; but we never had to. In four-and-a-half years we have proved to our satisfaction that the homœopathic methods work more rapidly, are cleaner, less painful and, in short, more satisfactory than the recognized orthodox ones. I have proved by a vast number of cases that this is so. Different types of cases which used to take weeks to get well under orthodox antiseptic treatment, recovered in just as many days as weeks previously. The staff increased naturally when more children returned to their old haunts; and the work has grown and the success of the homœopathic remedies has converted a number of nurses trained in orthodox hospitals.

The children on the whole must like our ways, they come regularly and are most disappointed if they do not get their little sweet pills, and they bring whole gangs of their friends and playmates for treatment. The experiment has been successful, as I thought it would be.

Arnica in potency is always given as soon as a child comes in suffering from the effects of an injury, fall, knock, cut, etc., even concussion, sprains, strains, bruising and so on, whether the case is slight or severe. They all get their dose of *Arnica*, which may have to be repeated half-hourly in a severe case, or only one dose is given in 24 hours for a slight injury. It always works astoundingly quickly in reducing the swellings, relieving the pain and shortening the period of shock and unconsciousness. *Arnica*, mother tincture 1 in 25—that is at the rate of one drop in 25 drops of water, is applied as an external dressing, provided there is no break in the skin, no abrasion, otherwise the Arnica will be absorbed and there is danger of *Arnica* poisoning, which resembles erysipelas. Therefore in the cases where the skin is broken, *Calendula* in the same strength as the *Arnica* is used as a routine measure and wonderfully quickly it acts, more rapidly than the hottest fomentation used to. It prevents sepsis, why it does it I do not know yet; the fact remains it does, unless an interfering parent, possessed of a little knowledge of first aid, chooses to remove the dressing applied at the clinic and uses his own favourite antiseptic; then we would find that the wound started to fester. I had to make myself very unpleasant to some of this tribe of "know-alls" in order to stop their game of interfering with our treatment. Let me repeat it, no iodine, no lysol or similar antiseptic, no boracic fomentations were used any more at the clinic; and, of course, no anti-tetanus injections were given, only plain, usually unboiled water and a few drops of either *Arnica, Hypericum* or *Calendula* tincture were used. If the wound or sore was already septic, *Hypericum* tincture in the same strength was ordered.

The district we worked in was heavily bombed, there was much rubble, much debris lying about, dirty bricks and stones and dust were scattered everywhere, hence an excellent breeding ground for septic germs and tetanus one would think. And yet no tetanus, no sepsis followed our revolutionary method which is absolutely opposed to the modern strict antiseptic treatment. These wide open spaces full of mounds of bricks, stones and twisted iron, full of gaping bomb holes, were exciting playgrounds for our young hopefuls, who imitated their fathers and elder brothers by fighting mock battles; only instead of guns, they used bricks and stones; injuries, often serious ones, are the results. And yet no sepsis followed if they came to us at once; and even infected wounds healed quickly under *Hypericum* locally combined with *Hypericum* in potency. Even injuries, of or near the eyes, contusions, etc., healed rapidly in a few days with *Arnica* internally and *Calendula* externally, although the eyes might be completely closed and the conjunctiva bloodshot at first; and so far I have not had any cases of cataract following these injuries. One of my workers who also attended a near-by eye hospital told me that in similar cases treated there, cataract was a frequent complication. I have seen and so have my nurses, enormous swellings disappear within a few hours, as if they had never existed and without leaving a trace, after *Arnica* internally and externally. If that happens where you can see the swelling and feel it on the outer surfaces of the body, is it not feasible that the same happens near an eyeball or inside the eye cavities? Anyway, the fact remains, no cataract has developed in these cases and I have seen the same youngsters and watched the eyes for months.

I regret we have no facilities for treating fractures, as there is no X-ray apparatus which is necessary to confirm the diagnosis. These cases are sent to hospital after a preliminary dose of *Arnica* for relief of pain and shock. In private work after an X-ray is taken, *Arnica* is given whenever required, the effusion of serum is reduced by a gentle soap and water massage, then a fixing apparatus, splint and bandage are applied after the fracture has been reduced and with daily light superficial massage and later ultra-violet treatment, passive and active movements of the muscles, the fracture heals rapidly. There is no reactionary rise of temperature or rise in the pulse rate at all, the patient sleeps well, the pain and shock is quickly relieved by repeated doses of *Arnica*. *Symphytum* in potency is prescribed after a few days in order to hasten the knitting together of the bone. In a multiple fracture of the olecranum where this treatment was applied, I got practically a full return of mobility at the injured elbow-joint in four weeks, as confirmed by a surgeon who was called for consultation, and no morphia was needed throughout.

Sprains and dislocations were treated with *Arnica* locally after they were reduced by gentle soap and water massage repeated daily. *Arnica* in potency was given as required, four-hourly at first, and I have seen a moderately severe sprained ankle with lacerated ligaments, recover completely in a week so that the patient was able to walk without any limp or disfiguring thickened ankle joint. Sometimes in milder cases the recovery was more rapid. If the bruising and contusion continued after the first day or two, the *Arnica* was discontinued and *Ledum* in potency, four-hourly, was given, and then the swelling and discoloration disappeared in a few days; 3-5 days were the maximum. A child jumped from a moving train on to the platform and injured one of the small bones of the foot. On X-ray examination three days later, a fracture was found. The parents gave *Arnica* at once and applied *Arnica* externally. The local doctor disapproved strongly and ordered lead lotion instead. I was rung up and ordered *Ledum* 6 at four-hourly intervals. When the dressing was taken off two days later by the local G.P., at the X-ray examination, she was surprised to find that there was no swelling and no discoloration of the foot and hardly any pain. All the comment the doctor made was: "You are lucky to get over it so rapidly."

A young farmer put the prongs of the pitchfork he used while manuring through the soft parts of his eyebrow and almost through his nose, he was badly shocked and almost blinded by the swelling. *Arnica* was given by his relatives at once. Ringing me up, I suggested *Ledum* in potency and *Calendula* lotion externally and ordered him to bed. He was well in 36 hours; the wound healed without any signs of sepsis, no tetanus followed, even though the fork was highly polluted with manure and the lock-jaw germs are usually found in highly manured soil. The old homœopaths advised *Ledum* as a prophylactic against lock-jaw; most doctors, even homœopaths, seem to prefer antitetanic serums in order to make doubly sure. Why? Have faith in your potencies and in your medicines; the germs are not any more potent now than they were 60 or 70 years ago, and the law holds good even against the most dreaded germs to this day.

If there is laceration of the superficial structures, torn skin and deep abrasions, even extending into the subcutaneous tissues, after giving two or three doses of *Arnica* to combat the preliminary shock, give *Hypericum* 1 in 10, later 1 in 25 as an external dressing. Do not remove that dressing, but keep moistening it with the diluted *Hypericum* whenever it appears dry to the touch. You will find very little or no sepsis; the surrounding inflammation will clear up in a few hours and the lacerated part will heal up in a few days. I have seen rapid cure of severe and extensive lacerations under *Hypericum*, while under the recognised methods of orthodox surgical treatment which I used to follow religiously for years, the severe injuries would take weeks to heal.

I am told on good authority that the Russian military surgeons in their campaigns use homœopathic methods almost exclusively in their advanced dressing stations, and their recovery rate is extraordinarily high, the patients return to the front line in a few days instead of weeks. The homœopathic treatment is so simple, so painless and the results are so rapid; more rapid than the modern sulphonamide and penicillin methods without any fear of serious constitutional disturbances or side effects coming on later. Some surgeons are already beginning to warn against the exclusive use of Sulphonamide pastes and ointments on septic wounds. And how soon will Penicillin be superseded?

For burns, too, homœopathic methods work exceedingly well.

In burns of the 2nd degree, give *Urtica Urens* 12th or 30th potency for the acute, agonising pain. I have timed it several times by a watch and found that the pain will be relieved in just about seven minutes without fail, repeat the dose, if it be required, whenever the pain returns, it may be in half an hour, one hour or two-four hours; or less often as required. It always acts rapidly. Locally apply *Urtica Urens* (1 in 10 or 1 in 25 as in all herbal lotions) on gauze dressings covering the whole burnt area; whenever the dressing appears to be dry, moisten the gauze with *Urtica Urens* lotion and cover it up with cotton wool and bandage. The patient, whenever the dressing gets uncomfortable, can usually be trusted to apply the lotion himself. Shock and pain disappear quickly and the healing takes place in a few days, even in extensive burns.

In burns of the 3rd degree, I have used *Causticum* 6, 12th or 30th potency, repeated as before whenever the pain returns. The relief of the pain was rapid, usually within seven-ten minutes. Externally, *Hypericum* lotion (1 in 10) should be applied and the dressing should not be disturbed unnecessarily, but should be moistened whenever it gets dry. The healing takes place in a much shorter time than under the orthodox methods. I saw a boy a year or two ago, who had an extensive 3rd degree burn of his right leg and abdomen, the right leg was treated by his parents with tannic acid jelly, before my arrival; the abdominal burn was overlooked. I applied *Hypericum* lotion to it; left the *Tannic Acid* alone until the next day, when it was changed to *Hypericum*. The abdominal burn was almost healed up in 24 hours, the burn on the thigh took four weeks! *Causticum* 30 relieved the pain and turned a shrieking, yelling child into a quiet one; in under ten minutes he was asleep. But the *Tannic Acid* made an awful mess of that right leg. The simple herbal lotions work much more efficaciously and with less pain and suffering.

In the most severe burns, especially when there is infection of the kidneys with dysuria, pain on passing water and passage of blood from the bladder and severe constitutional disturbances, *Cantharis* 6, 12, or 30, will deal with it effectively. It will heal up the local burn in a much shorter time than orthodox treatment can accomplish and the renal and bladder infection will be cured in a short time. You see, *Cantharis* is homœopathic or similar to this condition, that is, it produces a similar condition, disturbance of the genito-urinary tract with pain and frequency of micturition with passage of blood in the normal healthy prover, and therefore it cures this same condition if it is found in the sick. Try and prove it yourself. I have found it was the truth and nothing but the truth.

Many cases of death after severe and extensive burns with constitutional shock could be saved, if these simple rules were carried out.

A nursing sister burnt her face and eyes severely when a bottle of pure lysol exploded. *Hypericum* dressings were applied locally and *Causticum* 30 given hourly, less often when improvement sets in. She was back at her job in the surgery the next day with hardly any marks showing on her face except a slight redness; the eye showed no ill effects at all.

I recall a similar case seen many years go, when a colleague of mine burnt her right arm with pure lysol. She was badly shocked, and was off duty for nearly a fortnight, and the arm was badly scarred. Naturally, I was alarmed when I saw the condition of the Sister in the Dispensary staff, as I remembered vividly the other case; my case treated homœopathically got well in a few hours, even though it affected a much more vital part (eyes and face), while the other case treated by a well-known hospital surgeon, took weeks. Such is the difference between homœopathy and orthodox methods.

Let me impress upon you that I only teach and preach what I have seen myself; it is not hearsay, nor is it exaggeration, but plain unvarnished truth and clinical proof.

GUNPOWDER AS A PROPHYLAXIS OF SEPSIS

DR. CLARKE wrote a monograph on Gunpowder in 1915, from which the following is an extract:

Black gunpowder was discovered by the Alchemist Friar, Roger Bacon, and like a good many other things, it can cure as well as kill.

It comprises Sulphur, Carbon and Nitre, or Saltpetre, and the combination of these three powerful, well-known homœopathic medicines is also a remedy of great potency. It was well known by the North American Indians as a remedy in poisonous snake bites.

Our soldiers in the past century knew of it, and used it as a remedy for certain kinds of suppuration; they took it crude, mixed in hot water in teaspoonful doses.

The story goes that a Rector in East Anglia noticed that at the time of paring the sheep's feet, when suffering from foot-rot, his shepherds were always infected with blood-poisoning; the arm became swollen and black from the fingertips to the armpits, except in the case of one shepherd, who always escaped by dosing himself with black gunpowder mixed with cheese and eaten as a sandwich. The Rector was so struck with this preventive of the serious blood-poisoning which usually ended the career of a shepherd, so that he had to look around for another job—that he passed on the knowledge he had garnered; and blood-poisoning disappeared in his village.

Thus the great indication for the use of gunpowder is in *blood-poisoning*. It acts very well in minutes doses, in the homœopathic attenuations. It does not exert a direct germ-killing action; it acts by increasing the normal antiseptic action of the blood, and by raising the immunity. In health, living blood destroys germs; and the reason that in epidemics some persons escape the infection is that their blood is equal to destroying the germs which attack them. As has been explained previously, each substance, as it undergoes the process of graduated attenuation of the homœopathic pharmaceutical process, loses its physical properties and gains, on the other hand, the property of becoming radio-active. These attenuated substances are raised to a higher pitch of vibration and pass on these vibrations to the individuals who take them. Radium itself has the power of making each substance which comes in contact with its rays, *radiant,* and so the vibrations of the radio-active emanations are passed on.

Antiseptics are somewhat dangerous things; for if you want to kill the germs present in a wound, it is often necessary to apply antiseptics in such strength that the living cells of the body are damaged, and the vitality of the part is lowered. This is the reason for the slow healing of some wounds under the most careful antiseptic treatment. And therefore, it is of much importance to raise the vitality and resistance of the blood to the invading army of hostile germs. This can best be done by the action of the indicated remedy, and in cases of blood-poisoning, septic cuts and sores, septic eruptions, etc., it is the black *Gunpowder* in the 3rd decimal attenuation, that is in $\frac{1}{1000}$ grain doses, in which it acts promptly and painlessly.

For local dressings, after carefully cleansing the injured or septic parts with boiled water and clean sterilized lint, use tincture of *Calendula* or Common Marigold—or tincture of Witch Hazel (*Hamamelis*), in the proportion of one teaspoonful to the half-pint.

Dr. Clarke proved black gunpowder on himself by taking it in the 2*x* potency ; that is in $\frac{1}{100}$ grain doses, and produced severe facial herpes involving the right side of the nose, and the right eyebrow. So if you see a case of herpes of right eyebrow and nose, Gunpowder in minute attenuations (3*x* or 6*x*) will cure it for certain.

Gunpowder 3*x* is a perfectly safe domestic remedy, and should be better known among the public. Abrasions from falls would not turn septic, if cleansed carefully with boiled water and a tablet of *Gunpowder* was given three or four times a day for two or three days. It is thus a prophylactic, and will give protection against harmful germs; this method is much better than burning the skin with the strong tincture of iodine. In poisoned gnat bites, too, *Gunpowder* 3*x* three times a day rapidly cures the suppuration.

Thus far Dr. Clarke :

In the many minor septic conditions and sores of schoolchildren, I have used it with most gratifying results, acting on Dr. Clarke's advice.

I do not believe *Gunpowder* has ever had a proving in a woman, but this curious effect of Gunpowder was related by a woman patient; she was taking *Gunpowder* 3x on the advice of a homœopathic friend, I presume, for some minor septic condition, and she noticed that it increased the menstrual flow. The period was naturally scanty, and inclined to be painful; the freer the flow, the less pain there was. Since her discovery she has been taking *Gunpowder* 3x regularly, at the beginning of each period, and it invariably makes it flow more freely. The character of the period is very scanty; it begins, then stops for twelve hours, after which it comes on again; the *Gunpowder* 3x prevents this twelve-hourly intermission and increases the total quantity. She usually takes it at two-hourly intervals, and increases the interval as improvement takes place.

One was interested to get the following information : that among the working-class people, *Gunpowder* was well known and freely used as an abortifacient, naturally in crude doses; so it evidently has an expelling influence on the uterine mucous membrane.

Black Gunpowder when taken internally in small doses does not explode in *the body*, so there is no danger of any untoward action.

A METHOD OF TREATMENT OF FURUNCULOSIS

A BOIL or furuncle is a circumscribed form of necrosis of a small portion of skin and subcutaneous tissue round an inflamed hair follicle. It commences as a hard, tender, inflamed area with a central necrotic core which eventually bursts, discharging pus and subsequently the core or slough comes away; they are most frequently found under the axillae, on the forearms, glutei, face and chin and nape of the neck, where the friction of the collar may prolong the infection. Boils are frequently multiple and relapse is common. A carbuncle is a more extensive infective gangrene of the subcutaneous tissues due to a local invasion with pyogenic organisms, the commonest being the Staphylococcus aureus.

It begins as a hard, painful infiltration of the tissues, the skin over it becomes red and dusky. It spreads peripherally, the brawny centre portions become soft and boggy, and the skin shows signs of yielding to the pressure within. Vesicles and then pustules form on the surface which burst in turns, and ashy grey sloughs are discharged. Fresh openings develop gradually, the apertures enlarge and run into one another, producing a central irregular opening at the bottom of which lies the necrotic tissue. A large slough forms which gradually separates, leaving a clear granulating ulcer. Carbuncles most frequently occur on the shoulders, back, nates, and in men at the nape of the neck and the beard region.

There is sometimes considerable constitutional disturbance of an asthenic type; carbuncles on the face and upper lip especially may be followed by pyæmia or septicæmia, due to infective thrombosis of the cavernous sinus.

The infective organisms are Staphylococcus aureus, in rare cases S. albus, constipation, renal disease and diabetes predispose to the infection.

TREATMENT

During the last three years I have followed a new line of treatment, at first tentatively, combined with the usual surgical procedure, boric fomentation; and when pus has formed, an incision was made. Very soon I found that nothing beyond a dry dressing was required; and the furunculosis was rapidly aborted with the aid of a practically unknown remedy, derived from a Cuban spider. This spider, Mygale Cubensis or Cuban Tarentula, also found in Texas or South Carolina, is fairly large as spiders go, with a hairy, dark brown body. Its bite is painless, the person is not sensible of it until the next day, when an inflamed pimple is found, surrounded by a scarlet areola; from the pimple to some other part of the body a red erysipelatous line is seen, marking the line followed by the spider over the skin after biting. This pimple swells, the inflamed areola spreads, chills and fever set in with copious sweat and sometimes also retention of urine; the pimple becomes a hard, large, exceedingly painful abscess, ending with necrosis of the integuments over it and having several small openings, discharging a thick sanious matter containing pieces of necrosed cellular tissue; fascias and tendons; the openings by growing run into one another, forming a large cavity. At this period the fever takes on the intermittent type with evening exacerbations. In delicate children, the bite may prove fatal, but the majority recover in from three to six weeks.

The bite of this spider is followed by a carbuncle with more or less severe constitutional disturbances. Therefore according to the school of thought which bases its treatment on the Paracelsian axiom, "Similia Similibus Curentur," or "like cures likes," the substance which produced a carbuncle in the healthy individual should heal boils or carbuncles, produced by other means, provided you give it in small enough doses. Ocular proof of this theory of curing diseases by the like substances is not always easy to find; the symptoms produced by a drug are usually subjective and individual, and could be styled imaginary and therefore laughed out of court. But a boil following the bite of the Cuban spider is objective, and if the *Tarentula* given in small enough doses removes or cures a boil, this would be a positive proof of the correctness of the theory: "like cures like".

The following clinical cases may serve to illustrate this:

(1) Miss A.B., a young nursery governess, aged 21, otherwise healthy, presented a boil, size of a tangerine orange, in her left antecubital fossa, which had been slowly coming up for several days. It was fluctuating, an incision was made under local Ethyl Chloride, and a fomentation applied. *Tarentula cubensis* 30th

dilution was given at once, to be repeated three times a day. She lived some distance out of town and could not pay another visit for four days, I was somewhat doubtful what the outcome would be. The result was far beyond my expectations. In the specified time she returned and showed an arm entirely healed, the incision scar had healed, as if by first intention. There was no other sign of the boil, no discharge, no inflammation. She reported she felt better within ten minutes of leaving the surgery, and the discharge had dried up within less than twenty-four hours. She was mistress in a residential school, and there had been at that time several cases of furunculosis among the inmates; but none of the others had cleared up so rapidly.

(2) A boy, aged 10 years, was seen with a large carbuncle on his scrotum; he was almost bent double with the pain and dragging sensation in the scrotal sac and unable to sit down. The swelling was very hard, very tender and red; there was no fluctuation, and no testicles could be made out. His parents had already applied hot fomentations for days with little relief. He was ordered hot dry dressings, a suspensory bandage and *Tarentula cubensis* four-hourly. The nurse reported two days later that the swelling in the scrotum had disappeared: no sign of any carbuncle was discovered.

(3) Another boy, aged 12 years, had a boil, the size of a golf ball, in the abdominal wall over the left hypochondrium: fluctuation was present; but encouraged by the two previous cases, just mentioned, no surgery was attempted, dry dressings only were applied, and *Tarentula* given three times a day; two days later the boil had disappeared without causing any constitutional disturbance.

(4) A young woman, aged 25 years, developed several boils during the puerperium in the ward, and was discharged after three weeks with a high temperature, etc., in the care of a district nurse, owing to the shortage of beds. Temperature 102.8°, large boil in the right forearm, another forming on the left arm; looked very ill. *Tarentula cub.*, four-hourly. Temperature dropped in twenty-four hours and the furuncles retrogressed as usual under the remedy in two or three days; and four days after being first seen, she felt well enough to go for convalescence to the seaside; when seen a month later, she had completely recovered.

(5) W.E., a young commercial traveller, aged 26 years, was

seriously incommoded by recurrent boils for three months. He had eighteen boils during that time and considered going in for a course of vaccine. Persuaded to try *Tarentula cubensis*, three times a day instead. Reported a week later, the last and largest boil had dried up within forty-eight hours of starting treatment; and there was no further relapse for two years afterwards.

(6) A woman in the late forties developed a large, extremely painful boil in the groin and another on the perineum: whether this was a Bartholinian abscess or not, was never clearly made out, as she would not be examined at the time. *Tarentula cub.*, four-hourly; thirty-six hours later the boil on the perineum opened suddenly and discharged freely; three days afterwards both boils had disappeared.

Altogether this series included forty-eight cases of carbuncles and boils of varying sizes and in different positions: and all ages and both sexes with the following results:

Three cases were incised with Ethyl Chloride locally, one boil was on the left forearm, one was on the nape of the neck, and the third, a large axillary boil; they cleared up and were absolutely dry in two or three days with ten to twelve doses of *Tarentula cubensis*. No packing was required, no antiseptic dressings were used. The other forty-five cases had no surgical treatment; one depended entirely on the action of the *Tarentula* with mild local treatment, such as dry hot dressings. Invariably the result was: the inflammation subsided, and the boil or carbuncle aborted within forty-eight hours; a very large one might take three days. There was never any sign of septic infection left, no hardening of the tissues remained.

Three cases had some slight recurrence within the month; these were cases of furuncles of the nape of the neck, caused by acne, two were in young women, and the third, a lad of 13 years of age. The *Tarentula* was repeated, and the condition cleared up finally. The advantages of this method of treatment are psychological as well as economic: there is no surgical treatment, and therefore no pain, no discomfort, no fear of the knife, psychological peace.

Economical advantage is: one saves antiseptics, dressings, and the surgeon's and the nurse's time.

The series may be only small, but the results have been universally good, so that publication was deemed necessary.

The *Tarentula cubensis* can be obtained from any good homœo-pathic chemist, in the suitable dilution.

It should be stored in a dark cupboard, well away from all strong-smelling medicaments, such as camphor in any shape or form, menthol, etc., or the drug will become inactive, and no results will be obtained. This applies, of course, to all homœo-pathic medicines of whatever strength.

Since writing the above, I met a case of mammary abscess, involving the whole of the outer half of the left mammae, during lactation. The abscess was very hard, and tender, she could not bear to put the child to the breast, it had been gradually forming for a week; twenty-four hours' treatment with *Tarentula* local-ized the abscess, removed the pain and a small incision was made just outside the areola, where the abscess was pointing. Half an ounce of pus was removed, an external dressing of *Calendula* lotion was applied, the breast was lightly supported with a pad and bandage, and in another twenty-four hours the discharge had almost ceased; three days later the sinus had completely closed, and the mother was feeding again normally from that breast. *Silica* 6x, two-hourly, was given, after the abscess was opened, as experience had taught us that Silica assists in drying up a discharging sinus.

Still more experiences showing the advantage of Homœopathy over ordinary treatment in septic troubles.

A middle-aged man who thought he knew something about "septic fingers" and whitlows, had been treating a whitlow of his right thumb for two weeks with fomentations, Epsom salt dress-ings, soaking his thumb, etc., which made it rather worse. In des-peration he came to the dispensary: the thumb was cleaned up and dressed with mercurial lotion, the nail was gently lifted up, and the pus underneath released. He was treated for five days with very little improvement. Then he was seen by the Medical Officer who ordered *Silica* 30 three times a day; but made no other change. He showed himself again after two days, and the swell-ing of the thumb had gone down to normal, the sinus underneath the nail had dried up. Two days later the whole septic condition had disappeared, and the nail did not require to be taken off, as it was feared at first. Four days' treatment with homœopathic *Silica* in a high potency, and a septic nail healed up which had refused to do so for the three weeks previous to it. This is no miracle to the homœopathic surgeon, who sees such cases daily.

What a boon homœopathic treatment would be to the working man! Many weeks of treatment would be saved. Stiff fingers would be prevented, and there would be fewer compensation cases.

One remembers—this was years ago—a case of septic tenosynovitis and cellulitis of the right thumb going up the arm in a horse-keeper who had been bitten by a horse. *Hypericum* dressings and *Hypericum* 30, four-hourly, so changed this dangerous condition that he was discharged cured with a sound, freely movable thumb in less than a week.

I should not like to do without Homœopathy in the most serious septic conditions. I should guarantee a more rapid cure without antiseptics; notwithstanding the most virulent bacteria or even if antiseptics have to be used, supplement the local treatment with the indicated homœopathic remedy, and the cure will be much quicker.

Get hold of Carleton's *Homœopathy in Medicine and Surgery*. He gives clinical cases and indications for remedies in a variety of surgical cases.

PYROGEN (AFTER DR. GEORGE BURFORD)

THE remedies *Pyrogen* and *Septicaemin* are very little known and yet they are of such sovereign value that one can only regret that they do not stand in the front rank of homœopathic use and wont in the choice of the prescribers who act on the principle of the adjustment of remedy to malady.

Professor Burdon Sanderson was a great orthodox Materia Medica man and physiologist. He taught that decomposing organic materials were unique in inducing rise of temperature in the body. He did not go any further than that. Dr. Drysdale, a Homœopath, recognized the value of and began to experiment with this pyrexia-producing fluid on homœopathic lines as a powerful remedial measure. He called this crude substance used by him, *Pyrogen*, which he prepared by macerating raw beef in cold water, thereafter exposing this infusion for weeks to the rays of the sun. Burnett standardized this preparation and made use of it in fevers and blood-poisoning, the result of which he published in a monograph in 1888. The crude substance from which potencies were prepared in the usual manner was decomposing animal fluid, the retrograde change in its composition occurred outside the body. The American Homœopaths then began to make use of the septic substance of the morbid fluids of the body and proved then the close parallelism of the symptoms produced by the morbid agent and clinical human pathology.

Dr. Swan, who was the high priest and instigator of the high dilution school, raised the morbid *Pyrogen* containing material from the contents of a septic abscess to the highest level of transcendental potencies, and commenced that series of well-nigh miraculous cures which are only paralleled by the clinical experiences of Hahnemann himself in the post-Napoleonic years. These potencies of Swan were made from septic pus; Sherbino later made provings with Swan's potencies: while the earlier British work was done with decomposing beef as the crude primary agent, but the therapeutic successes were astounding whether made, as in America, with septic pus, or as in England, with septic beef. As time went on, the tendency was to change the potency from 6*c*., administered night and morning, to 10 *m*. or *cm*., administered in unit doses.

CLINICAL EXPERIENCES

Burnett used mainly the 6th centesimal dilution two-hourly in acute cases.

Shuldham employed the same potency in two cases of diphtheritic sore throat.

Sherbino cured a case of puerperal fever and was led to its selection by the high pulse rate.

Hunt cured with *Pyrogen* 200 an elderly woman suffering for years with an ulcerated leg riddled with deep burrowing ulcers.

And Swan gives as a special indication for *Pyrogen*, pulse abnormally rapid and out of proportion to the temperature.

The principal symptoms are :

Disproportion between pulse and temperature; pulse continually rises.

Restlessness owing to soreness of parts.

Better sitting up in bed and in the act of rising, relieved by stretching out limbs, hands and arms are numb : great benefit from heat and movement.

One of my earliest experiences of the great benefit of *Pyrogen* on the suffering individual was in Dr. Burford's wards. This woman had had an extensive and serious operation. I think it was a fallopian tube abscess followed by peritonitis. She recovered well after various homœopathic remedies, but there was extensive sloughing of the abdominal wound which would not heal, along with a fistula leading to an opening into the peritoneal cavity. There was pyrexia around about 99° and 100° and pulse rate of 150. Dr. Burford with his clinical acumen suggested to me the making of an auto-vaccine from the patient's own pus, and I was entrusted with the making of this auto-pyrogen according to homœopathic rules. I chose several bottles, macerated a platinum loopful of the pus from the abdominal wound as far down as I could go with the probe—and then took one drop of this macerated pus and mixed it with 99 drops of rectified spirit. This was in 1913 and rectified spirit was cheap and in general use in homœopathic hospitals. Then I succussed this dilution and labelled it 1*c*.; then I took one drop of this dilution and mixed it with 99 drops of rectified spirit, succussed it well and labelled it 2c., and repeated this process carefully six times in all, until I had the 6c. dilution. Of this 6c. potency the patient had five drops night and morning, and in less than a week the wound had healed up from the bottom and the scar was sound and firm. One remembers how pleased Dr. Burford was with the result; the patient was seen three months later and showed a strong scar with no signs of a threatening hernia. It made a deep impression on one's mind, especially as one recalled a similar case in the wards of Edinburgh Infirmary in a middle-aged man of 55 who had extensive suppuration of the abdominal wound and a sinus leading down to peritonium after an operation for a ruptured duodenal abscess, and he was round about six months in the wards before this wound healed up. And the patient in the Homœopathic Hospital treated with *Pyrogen* was out after a month or barely five weeks. An astonishing difference! No wonder that one thought highly of the power of *Pyrogen* in septic cases. As Dr. Burford puts it succinctly : *ubi venenum, ibi remedium*—where the poison is, there is the remedy, the cause may also evoke the cure.

Some further examples of the use of *Pyrogen* in dangerous cases may show its extreme value in emergencies.

During the serious influenza epidemic in 1918-19, one's clinical acumen was greatly tried, but again and again one was thankful for the very efficient aid that homœopathic medicines provided, and over and over again an apparently serious case quickly turned the corner.

Patients used to say, "I only had a very mild case of 'flu." They never gave the credit of the rapid cure to the almost tasteless watery medicines they used to imbibe. There were no complications, no heart trouble, no broncho-pneumonia, no septic pneumonias, and therefore no fatal incidents in over a hundred cases. A triumph for Homœopathy indeed. Very few cases gave me much anxiety. The only relapse I had was a lady dispenser who knew so much that she wished to almost treat herself, and she had several weeks in bed and was far more pulled down afterwards than any of the other cases, even though she had the same strict starvation diet, copious draughts of barley water, lemon juice, orange juice and grapes as the other patients I looked after. So I proved to myself that a natural diet, a fruitarian diet alone, was not the greatest factor in promoting a rapid cure. It always wanted the indicated—that is the right homœopathic remedy—for each individual case.

There was another case that caused me some anxiety, as it would not respond to the usual remedies. He was a young man invalided out of the army on account of shrapnel wounds in his ankle. The rest of his family, both parents, several brothers and sisters, responded quickly to the treatment given, temperatures came down within twelve to twenty-four hours. They were kept in bed for seven days, after the first day of normal temperature, and kept for two or three days only on a fruit diet which was gradually augmented by ordering vegetable soups and egg dishes. His mother could not understand why her eldest son did not get well as quickly as the rest, and put it down to the effects of the war wounds. She was not far wrong either, as it turned out in the end. After nearly a week of pyrexia I had visited him at all hours of the day and night to get all the symptoms collected together, nurses were at a premium just at that time, and one depended on the relatives, provided there was anybody left to do the nursing, and I carried several door keys in my pockets to let myself into the various houses. Well, eventually I got the following disease picture : very high, steadily rising temperature, going up to 105° at night, the pulse remaining somewhere about 100-110, therefore the pulse and temperature were quite out of proportion. He was extremely restless, never staying long in one position, very confused as regards the number of extremities he owned, there seemed to be so many arms and legs in the bed; he complained of the extreme hardness of the bed, his back was so painful and the bed was as hard as a board. He had received *Rhus. tox.* for his restlessness, also *Arnica* for the hardness of the bed and (?) remote effects of war injuries; also *Baptisia*, which seemed to correspond to the confusion of the mind and the sensation of there being more than one person in the bed; nothing would touch the illness, however; the weakness went from bad to worse. There were drenching sweats, an offensive, penetrating odour from his perspiration; he had to change his shirts several times in the twenty-four hours; his mouth and tongue were foul, and yet *Mercury* did not touch him. I did not give up hope, but continued to study the case. In the back of my mind I knew there was something that would act as a key to open the door to this maze, this complicated septic fever. Suddenly it came to me, there was a certain remedy which had this arrhythmia of pulse

and temperature, a high temperature with a low pulse or vice
versa. This was *Pyrogen*, and in reading up *Pyrogen* in the
Materia Medica, there was the simillimum; the extreme restlessness, the bruised feeling of the parts lain on, the relief by movement of feet, by change of position; offensive, disgusting perspiration, great weakness and lassitude: it was all there. So *Pyrogen
cm.*—the only potency I had except the *mm.*, both Heath Potencies from America—was given two-hourly in a watery solution,
and by the morning, a few hours after the late night visit—I found
the patient had slept more restfully and the temperature was
down to 100°, that night, within twenty-four hours of starting
this new medicine, the temperature was normal, and it kept
normal after that. I continued the remedy for a couple of days
and then finished off with one dose of *Pyrogen mm.*, dry on the
tongue. I do not remember now, whether he had a constitutional
remedy at the end of "seven days bed," after the temperature
reached the normal level. Anyway, the patient was kept under
observation for several years afterwards, and he had no after-
effects from his serious attack of "wartime 'flu," and on the
whole he came off quite lightly, compared with many other
victims; he was only in bed for a little over two weeks: eight
days' temperature and seven days' recuperative rest. In this case
normal influenza, if one may be allowed to call any influenza
normal—was complicated by previous inoculations of the various
typhoid, paratyphoid and cholera bacilli; he had had anti-
malarial inoculation, he had been vaccinated, he had anti-
streptococcal injections and inoculations against tetanus, and he
could not remember what other inoculations he had had to sub-
mit to. I came to the conclusion that he was full of septic matter,
and his blood stream was a battlefield of all sorts of serums and
bacteria, and hence the drenching sweats, the high temperature,
the offensive odour and the extreme prostration.

In my own mind I am absolutely convinced that this young
man would have been another of the numerous victims of the
fatal influenza epidemic, if it had not been for our *Pyrogen*.

A number of years passed by, but the lesson one was taught of
the action of *Pyrogen* was never forgotten. One day I heard of a
poor woman lying dangerously ill in her own home after her
confinement: she had been in hospital antenatally for several
weeks with high temperature due to pyelitis, the story went, and
was sent out even though the fever, etc., had not abated, under

the care of a district nurse with the instruction to call in a local doctor. There was such a call on the hospital beds, she had to be discharged. I heard of her accidentally, she had been at home for nearly a week since her return from hospital : the visitor told me that the temperature would not come down, but stayed round about 103°, the pulse was only about 80 though; she was so weak she could not look after her baby, a kind neighbour was seeing to it. It seemed so tragic, poor Mrs. D. being so ill, as there was a large family of seven or eight children.

Across my mind flashed the story of the soldier suffering from septic influenza and his cure by *Pyrogen*; here, once again, was the abnormal pulse-temperature ratio. As there was no doctor in attendance, the woman was too poor to pay for one, and the nurse was so worried, a dozen powders of *Pyrogen* 30 were sent, with the instructions to take one powder at four-hourly intervals, with the result that the evening temperature, the first temperature taken after the powders had been sent, was 99.8°, and the next morning the temperature was normal and stayed normal.

The patient reported herself a couple of weeks later as being very well except for a crop of vesicles on both her wrists and hand, which cleared up with a dose of *Sulphur* 30. Here, once again, was a septic fever, caused by, and following on, some infection of the female generative organs, cured by *Pyrogen*, which eliminated the poison, as often happens after homœopathic medication, through the skin.

A little while ago I came across this abnormal pulse-temperature ratio in a case of post-operative pyrexia. *Pyrogen* was exhibited and pulse and temperature came down together and the patient reported the curious fact that shortly after taking the powder she could taste pus in her throat and mouth. She was a vegetarian and had never tasted meat in her life, so she said, and was probably hypersensitive. I gave her unmedicated powders to try and prove the veracity of her statements; and she only complained of the putrid taste after a *Pyrogen* powder. As it was given in the 30th potency, it was certainly not a physiological reaction, more in the form of a proving.

Pyrogen—which is a product of sepsis—cures septic fevers of all kinds and conditions when the symptoms agree; it was proved on healthy individuals, and produced a distinctive type of pyrexia with definite clear-cut indications. Thus it proves again the great truth of the Homœopathic Law : *Like cures like.* In my hands it cured septic influenza, puerperal pyelitis, and post-operative pyrexia, and it will continue to cure other septic diseases showing the typical symptoms.

Many cases of blood-poisoning and ptomaine poisoning, peritonitis, and pyæmia could be saved by *Pyrogen*, if the medical practitioners would only study our Materia Medica and apply it in cases which show the characteristics I mentioned. *Pyrogen* is closely related to various other remedies, it is very similar to *Rhus. tox.*, to *Baptisia*, to *Arnica;* one has to get together all the distinctive symptoms of each case and then apply the simillimum, the remedy which is most similar. The general medical profession is getting an inkling of the truth, as it is using the serum and vaccines made from individual bacteria or a combination of bacteria, found in different septic cases and injecting them hypodermically, and in certain cases they do get a positive reaction, a good curative result. But their doses are too big, and the results are too uncertain, and until they learn to give minute doses and apply them according to a definite law of cure, their results will never be as good as our remedies applied strictly, following the laws discovered by Hahnemann:

(1) The single remedy.

(2) The minute dose.

(3) Given on the totality of the symptoms found in the individual patient, and corresponding to the symptoms produced by healthy provers.

An interesting confirmation of the value of *Pyrogen* in preventing blood-poisoning comes from a keen homœopathic layman who worked in Smithfield meat market. He found that *Pyrogen* taken immediately after being scratched, when handling carcases of meat which were frequently not any too sound, stopped any infection occurring. He used to distribute *Pyrogen* 30 to his friends after septic scratches on arms and hands from handling septic meat, and invariably cured these lesions. He was very enthusiastic about the magic that rested in the minute doses of *Pyrogen*, and here the homœopathic law proved itself again as being correct. The septic meat produced septic scratches and inflammation ascending up the arm, and *Pyrogen*, septic meat in homœopathic doses, cured it.

Magna est Veritas et praevalebit!

NARCOLEPSY

(Irresistible Sleepiness)

"Suddenly she fell asleep." The daily papers are always out after medical curiosities, and have been making a front page incident of a young woman in the early twenties who falls asleep every time she laughs. She went to the pictures, laughed at the jokes, fell asleep suddenly and could not be awakened, so that she had to be taken home in an ambulance, and then slept for four hours. Any sudden shock affected her in the same way, it might be anger or laughter. This mental disorder has recently been classified by Dr. Adie, who, since 1926, examined some fifty cases in the following four years, and described this affliction, which he called narcolepsy, under the following terms. "It is character-ized by attacks of irresistible sleep without apparent cause, and curious attacks of emotion, in which the muscles relax suddenly, so that the victim falls to the ground, often fully conscious, and yet unable to move." There are two different kinds of attacks :

(1) Sleep attacks. Spontaneous seizures, the patient remains more or less unconscious.

(2) Catalepsy. This is caused by violent emotion, anger, joy, laughter—therefore truly a case of helpless laughter. He becomes stiff and helpless, knows what happens, but can't help himself and does not always lose consciousness. This condition may come on after a period of stress and strain, for example when a patient has not been having sufficient sleep for a considerable time. The sufferer gets "sleepy attacks" during the daytime at first, especi-ally after eating, such as after heavy lunches in the middle of the day, when the brain is naturally anæmic, nearly all the blood being required for the process of digestion. The sleep lasts from fifteen to twenty minutes, and in no way differs from ordinary sleep. On the Continent the siesta after the mid-day meal is encouraged rather than otherwise, and the German calls this post-prandial somnolence *nur ein Viertelstündchen*. These sleepy attacks are liable to come on at such times, when normal people feel sleepy, only in a more exaggerated form, say in a hot close

room or in an overheated railway compartment during a long journey. The normal person can be roused, but the narcoleptic cannot.

The usual professional advice is not to fight against this irresistible desire for sleep, but to give way to it and have a short nap. Again, it has been noted that narcoleptics fall asleep the moment they get into bed and sleep well and long.

A cataleptic attack is usually caused by laughter. Everything goes limp, the knees give way, the arms drop to the side, the eyelids close and the patient falls to the ground, helpless, unable to speak, but well aware of everything that goes on around him. Such an attack, it is stated, can be warded off by not giving way to emotion, to anger or to laughter. What a dull life! not even to be allowed to laugh at Mickey Mouse or the antics of Charlie Chaplin!

This condition of narcolepsy, even though apparently quite a new disorder, and which has only recently been fully studied and classified by the medical scientist, must have been met with years ago, for that keen observer of human nature and its frailties—Charles Dickens—gives a good description of a narcoleptic in the fat boy of Dingley Dell in the *Pickwick Papers*. This boy would drop off to sleep at the most unexpected moments, while standing and serving at table, while sitting in the front seat of a coach, in the very act of knocking for admission at a door, he would go to sleep. He fell into a deep sleep even during meal times, while indulging in the very heavy repasts which Dickens relates with such loving detail. Narcolepsy is therefore not a modern disease. It was known to the homœopathic physicians as well, for in the large *Repertory* of Kent, that symposium of numerous exact symptoms, a column and a half is devoted, not to narcolepsy or catalepsy (these scientific names have only recently been coined), but to the simple term "falling asleep," which does neither daze nor mystify, but is good plain English and can be understood by all and sundry. There are separate items for falling asleep in the morning, noontide while eating, afternoons while sitting, evenings after eating, and so on.

For the information of the colonial readers and others interested who are far away from the ken of a homœopathic physician, I shall give some of these rubrics and the remedies from Kent's *Repertory*, fourth edition:

Falling asleep, mornings : Coca., hep., lyc.

,, forenoons : Calc.

,,   ,, while reading : Nat. sulph.

,, noon : Aloe.

,,   ,, while eating : Puls.

,, afternoon : Bar. Carb., cina, dios., hyos., mag. c., nat. m., phys., sabad., sep.

,,   ,, while sitting : Nat. mur.

,, evenings : Ammon. carb., mez.

,,   ,, after eating : Ammon. carb., gels.

,, while reading : Mez.

,, while sitting : Apis, hep., Nux vom., tell.

,, 5 p.m., while sitting : Nat. mur.

,, when answering : Arn., Bapt., hyos.

> (N.B.—You find this state in serious cases of pyrexia, such as typhoid, intermittent fevers, tropical fevers, influenza, etc.)

,, after beer : Thea.

,, breakfast : Sumbul.

,, during conversation : Caust., tarax.

,, after dinner : Ant. t., caust., coca., cur., *Mag. carb.*, tabacum.

,, after eating : Arum tig., bor., calc. p., gamb., lyc., mur. ac., nat. m.

,, during heats : *Ant. t.*, *apis.*, Calad., Eup. per., gels., ign., Lach., lyc., Mez., Nat. mur., Nux m., Op., Podo., Rob., Samb., stram.

,, after laughing : Phos.

> (N.B.—You see this curious condition of "falling asleep after laughing" was known to the early Homœopaths, and unless there are other symptoms contra-indicating *Phos.*—*phos.* should cure narcolepsy after laughing.)

,, from the least mental exertion : Ars., chloral., ferr., Hyos., ign., kali. br., *kali c.*, nat. s., *nux v.*, tarax.

,, after pain : Phyt.

,, while reading : Angustura, cimic., *colch.*, ign., iris, lyc., mez., *nat. m.*, nat. s., plat., ruta, sep.

,, while sewing : Ferrum.

,, while sitting : Acon., ang., ant. t., apis, ars., arum t., aur., calc. p., china, cimic., *cina*, ferr., form., hep., ign., kali. br., kali. carb., lyc., merc., muriatic acid, nat. c., *nat. m.*, nat. p., NUX VOM., puls., *sep.*, tell., thuj., tarent.

„ while standing : Acon., corr. r., mag. c., morph.

„ after dinner : Mag. c.

„ after stool : *Æth.*, elaps., *sulph.*

„ while talking : Caust., *chel.*, mag. c., morph., ph. ac.

„ after vomiting : *Æth.*, bell. (N.B.—"This precious little symptom, falling asleep after vomiting, has saved many a life in very acute cases of infantile diarrhœa and vomiting.")

„ from weakness : Petr., phos.

„ after wine : Thea (also after beer).

„ while writing : Phos. ac., thuja.

You see, this gives quite a full and detailed account of what are or might be the concomitant symptoms of "sudden dropping asleep."

For example, if I had been asked to do something for the fat boy in *Pickwick Papers*, I should have taken the rubrics : after dinner, while standing, while standing after dinner, while talking, while talking after dinner—and the remedy working through all this would be *Mag. carb.* I should then look up *Mag. carb.* in the Materia Medica books, and there one finds "inordinate craving for meat"—and there you are. I should expect to cure this "fat boy" of his sleepiness and over-eating and eventually of his obesity.

One remembers a case which happened years ago, long before narcolepsy and catalepsy were officially recognized, classified and differentiated. I diagnosed it then as an automatic state in a case of pituitary obesity. A young woman, very stout, big and pale, used to be suddenly seized with attacks of sleepiness, drowsiness and automatic behaviour during her menstrual periods.

She was an active, intelligent girl, a clerk, well thought of by her firm, who every month was suddenly taken like this. She became drowsy and dazed, and could not answer, stared stupidly when addressed, heard and saw everything, could remember everything afterwards, but was quite speechless and unable to move at the time. Everything seemed far off to her, she did not seem to recognize her friends even. I saw her once in this state, and very pitiful she looked. In between she was always bright, active and happy, though very worried about these peculiar attacks which invariably happened every month, during the periods. She was very much afraid of losing a good job, as she always had to have two or three days off. There were other symptoms present which led me to the right remedy : she complained of a dry mouth, the tongue literally stuck to the roof of her mouth, and yet she was never thirsty; she was flatulent, very constipated before and during her periods, the stool was soft, not hard as a constipated stool usually is, she felt the cold weather, especially the cold, damp weather, and yet hated a close, warm room, which always made her more sleepy and dazed. She fainted easily, when she had to stand, and then there was this automatic conduct, this sleepiness, drowsiness and confusion of mind. The only remedy that covered all these symptoms was *Nux moschata*, the common nutmeg. She was given *Nux moschata cm.*, the only potency I had got; for three months she had no return of her attacks, and these had been troubling her for two years at least; then another severe attack, during which I saw her, the first time I had actually seen her in an attack. Then another dose of *Nux moschata cm.* which held her for six months this time; she had only a slight return of her old trouble, then three doses of *Nux moschata*; and then no further medicine was required. The trouble ceased. The *Nux moschata* had helped her "to grow out of this affliction."

Two years afterwards I met her, a healthy, bonny-looking woman on the eve of getting married. Never had any trouble since. Lately I have lost sight of her, but she promised to come back, if there should be a return. In Homœopathy one does not depend on grand sounding names, and one falls back on the Materia Medica, on the symptoms laboriously collected by generations of conscientious provers, doctors and lay people, who put down in common everyday language their reactions after taking a remedy. We meet certain symptoms in a sick person, and we try to find the simillimum, the most like medicine; and after having found it, we confidently predict and expect a cure. We should give the poor, young, narcoleptic woman who is afraid of laughing for fear of bringing on an attack, the indicated remedy, basing our selection on the remedies found in the *Repertory* under the different headings; it would probably be *Phos.*, but it might be something else, and the result would be a happy normal individual, once more able to enjoy a joke to the full : no longer cut off from all fun and enjoyment.

BRONCHOPNEUMONIA

HOMŒOPATHS are said to be powerless against serious acute diseases; therefore let us see whether we can refute this statement of our opponents.

Bronchopneumonia, according to the text-books, is a terminal disease, which means, it comes along at the end of an illness and finishes it—fatally as a rule. More than 50 per cent. of cases of bronchopneumonia succumb to it, and it is therefore rightly feared in allopathic hospitals and under allopathic treatment. Now hear what a sister of one of the homœopathic hospitals said about this very same disease in her wards. She could not understand why there should be so much bother about bronchopneumonia, "they always get well in a few days in this hospital and we have no deaths." This is the testimony of a trained nurse, who sees behind the scenes and is therefore a good judge.

I have had much personal contact with bronchopneumonia in practice, I have seen the results of allopathic treatment in young children, it usually meant writing off the case as another fatality. On District I used to get the cases frequently from other doctors who had given up a particular child as being beyond hope, moribund in fact, and Homœopathy used to pull them round invariably.

Only one case of bronchopneumonia ended fatally. This was an infant, not a fortnight old, who developed a slight cold and slight cough; she was sent home with orders to be kept warm and with some medicine, one forgets what it was. The next day an almost impenetrable black sooty fog occurred all over London. And this foolish young mother took her infant out in this sulphurous atmosphere right across London. She was out several hours in this fog and had to walk most of the way, as there were no vehicles running; just in order to show the infant to its grandmother! Naturally, an acute attack of bronchopneumonia supervened, and this infant died twenty-four hours later; she was too young to withstand the large doses of sulphurous fog she had swallowed.

Now for an example of bronchopneumonia in a child. This was a child aged eighteen months, the only boy in a family of girls, and as the parents were middle-aged and not likely to have another, it was important to them that their only boy should live. He had been ill for over a week, and the local doctor had given up the case as the bronchopneumonia was too far gone; the child certainly looked moribund when I saw it. He was only semi-conscious; respirations over 60 per minute, temperature was 104°, pulse weak and thready, almost uncountable, round about 160; cold sweat was on his forehead; you could hear the laboured breathing from outside the door.

A most unpromising case : death was very close indeed. I tried *Antimonium tartaricum m.* in three-hourly doses, on the following symptoms : dilated, sooty nostrils which were flapping with each breath; lungs full up with mucus, impossible to raise the phlegm. Coarse rattling sounds in chest; great weakness, lack of reaction. There was no result, no change in twenty-four hours, and no response to *Antimonium tart.* Did I give up then and turn my back on this nearly dead child? Oh no, we had other weapons still at our call. There was *Lycopodium* which has al-most identical symptoms; I noticed that the right side of the lungs seemed worse, and the father said that trouble had started on the right side; also there was wrinkling of the forehead. We have to go in for such minutiae in homœopathic treatment which seems so unimportant to other doctors, and yet make all the difference between life and death sometimes. *Lycopodium* 1m., two-hourly, was prescribed, and to my joy the next time I went in, the respirations and the pulse had dropped—forty-eight hours after the first dose of *Lycopodium* had been given, the tempera-ture was normal, and within less than a week from my first visit the child was perfectly well, the lungs were clear and no signs of any bronchopneumonia were left. A triumph for Homœopathy; what magic rests in the correctly applied remedy !

I had many such cases; sometimes *Antomonium tartaricum* would perform the miracle, sometimes *Lycopodium* would act in the same way, *according to the symptoms* found; other times it was *Sulphur* which saved the situation; and very frequently again it was *Phosphorus*. One has to consider all the symptoms, and according to what were the predominating symptoms, the corres-ponding medicine was chosen, and confidently one could predict success: there were never any later complications. No emphysema followed, no unresolved patches of pneumonia were left behind. The cure followed quickly and gently after each correctly given remedy. I was present on one occasion at a discussion at an Invalid Children's Aid Association meeting on the very serious results of emphysema after bronchopneumonia, and the best steps to take to alleviate this evil. Apparently it cost this Association hundreds of pounds in money for convalescing these emphysematous children. And yet under homœopathic treatment you *do not see* these cases! Would it not be worth while if doctors studied some of these remedies I mentioned and gave them to these bronchopneumonic children? And even later when emphysema has developed, our remedies will clear it up. Kent's *Repertory* mentions thirty remedies under the rubric "Emphysema," so there is plenty of choice and the right remedy can be found, if each case is carefully studied and investigated. There is no need even to give the high potencies, the transcendental doses I mention: the lower potencies work, more slowly in my opinion; but they do work. Try the remedies in the 3rd decimal attenuations, and results will follow.

Now for another very interesting case of bronchopneumonia. A young lady, early thirties, was fighting a slight bronchial cold for about a week, and unfortunately at this stage, exigencies of her profession made it necessary for her to expose herself to the vagaries of this climate and go a long railway journey across country and stay for twenty-four hours in lodgings. She collapsed with a high temperature on her return home and had to stay in bed. As she was a good Homœopath, she took frequent doses of *Aconite* 3*x* to bring down the temperature, unfortunately she was beyond the aid of *Aconite*, and twenty-four hours later I was called in. I found a delirious patient with brilliantly flushed cheeks, respirations round about 28, pulse 128 and temperature 102.8°—constant dry cough with rusty, blood-stained mucus, which was difficult to bring up. Sharp cutting pains right base of lungs each time she moved, and whenever she coughed. On examination I found signs of bronchitis and friction sounds at the right base indicating the presence of pleurisy besides bronchitis. She was very thirsty, constantly drinking cold water, and then there were these sharp cutting pains in her side.

This seemed to spell *Bryonia*, and I left *Bryonia* 30 to be taken half-hourly while necessary, the intervals to be lengthened if the pains, etc., improved. I also ordered anti-phlogistine to be applied to the right side at the back and a firm bandage round the whole chest for support. Twenty-four hours later the condition was unchanged, pulse, respiration and temperature remained at the same level, only the acute stitching, cutting pains were improving. I continued to give *Bryonia* as before, which she had for three days altogether; it made no impression on the disease; it removed the pains, that was all. The dullness in the back extended higher up, crepitations were made out on the right side as high up as the apex of the scapula, and there were rhonchi and râles all over the lungs. Temperature remained round about and between 102° and 103°, the pulse was between 120 and 130, respirations between 28 and 30. Just a typical case of early broncho-pneumonia in a young well-developed adult after exposure.

After three days one reviewed the case and took the symptoms again. She was bringing up rusty, blood-stained sputum; there was a feeling of weight and heaviness and aching in her chest, great thirst for cold water, great aversion to tea, which she was very fond of as a rule; anxious delirium, she was subconsciously worrying as to whether it was time to take the horrid medicine again; was rather loquacious when she woke up; vivid delirious fancies on being aroused from sleep and on falling asleep. All this indicated *Phosphorus* now, and on the third day I gave her *Phosphorus* 3x in frequent doses, two-hourly, I think. She had very vivid fancies in her delirium, she thought the bed was crowded so that there was no room for the hot water bottle in the bed; there were too many people in the bed, she talked of three people being in bed with her. Fortunately I did not know this, or I might have given her a different medicine which would not have answered so well. The skin of her face was so tight, she had to put on cold cream to ease it; her lips were parched and dry and cracked. Twenty-four hours later, to my great astonishment, pulse and temperature were still the same, the symptoms were unaltered. What to do now? The remedy was still indicated, but the potency was wrong. I went higher and gave her *Phos.* 30, four-hourly. The next day the temperature was down to 101.2° and the pulse was 96 in the evening, twenty-four hours after the first dose of *Phosphorus* 30.

I was delighted at the response I got from *Phos.* 30 and continued to give it four-hourly. In another twenty-four hours the temperature was normal and the pulse down to 72. Within forty-eight hours of first giving *Phosphorus* in the 30th potency, the temperature dropped from 102.4° to normal, and the pulse came down from 128 to 72, and the respirations from 28 to 20. That was six days after the first visit.

Now for the subsequent history : the cough was still trouble-some, even though there was no more blood-stained sputum; this disappeared when *Phos.* 30 was first given; the dull patch of right-sided basal pneumonia cleared up completely within two weeks : that is, a week after the temperature had gone down, the patch disappeared. The bronchial sounds went four days after the temperature became normal. The patient was kept on water, grapes and dilute orange-juice while the temperature was up, and as the temperature came down she was allowed Brand's chicken essence and later Marmite, vegetable soup, brown bread and butter were added; and then three days after the temperature was down, a light chicken, vegetable and egg diet was permitted. She was kept on *Phos.* 30 for several days, and then after a week *Phos. xm.* was given, which completed the cure.

Let me repeat, this patient's temperature became normal on the seventh day of her illness within forty-eight hours after *Phos.* 30 had been given : the bronchitis and pneumonic patch cleared up *in toto* within twelve days. There was no cardiac weakness, the patient was clamouring to be up and about within three days after the temperature was normal, as she felt so well; but pru-dence prevailed, and she stayed in bed over a week after the normal temperature. "A mild case of bronchopneumonia" do I hear that mutter in the background?

Does even a mild case of bronchopneumonia recover so com-pletely in less than fourteen days? The effect of the *Phosphorus* was so prompt after it had been given that there was not the slightest doubt whatever that it was due to the *Phosphorus* that the improvement set in; but the curious way in which *Phos-phorus* 3x would not work, while *Phos.* high did its work so rapid-ly and smoothly. The patient was used to low potencies, so I thought I should give a low potency first. The general opinion among homœopathic physicians is "give a low or medium pot-ency in acute diseases" and "leave higher potencies to chronic diseases."

One has to find out in each patient which potency acts best. Begin with a low potency and stick to it, if you have faith in a low potency. If the symptoms remain the same and you have faith in your selection, you know your remedies and you know it cannot be another remedy, do not change it, but go higher, try 6x or 12x or 30x if you like and you find the higher potency will act, where the lower potency fails.

Kent's *Repertory* quotes seventeen remedies for pleuropneumonia (bronchopneumonia) and thirteen remedies for typhoid pneumonia, I am not sure whether he means pneumonia in the later stages of typhoid (the terminal bronchopneumonia of the orthodox school) or just bronchopneumonia with accompanying weakness, as you would find it in the typhoid. As I said before it is a question of studying your patient, watching and observing all the minute symptoms—having a good nurse at hand, who can report all the little details which occur during your absence, and then putting it all together and finding the counterpart among the remedies given in the *Repertory*.

Nash's *Leaders in Homœopathic Therapeutics* gives very good pictures of remedies which are easily recognized, even by the tyro.

Allen's *Keynote of Leading Remedies* is another useful book for the beginner. During a conversation I had with a German doctor working in a homœopathic drug-house, we discussed the merits of various homœopathic books; he agreed with me that Nash's *Leaders* was a very good Materia Medica book for the beginner, except that the high potencies, he declared, were moonshine. That was the opinion of a low potency man, and in Germany, I fancy, judging from their publications, it appears they only give low potencies. This is very curious, for the master in Homœopathy, our Hahnemann, was after all a German, and he gave up the lower potencies in his later years in favour of the higher ones. The reason he gave for this change was that there was less aggravation after a high potency than after a low one. Are the present race of German doctors more material than the great Hahnemann? He was after all a great philosopher and metaphysician, and the German race has produced many great philosophers in the past. It seems strange that the much more practical and material American race should produce the high potency men, and that an idealistic philosophical people, such as the Germans, should cling to the more material doses. High potencies act, and act rapidly, but they have to handled with care. It is much better to stick to the lower potencies, unless you know your Materia Medica very well. Also high potencies have to be very carefully made, must be stored properly, or they lose their virtue rapidly. Therefore they should not be sold or stocked by chemists on the same shelves with other strong-smelling crude drugs such as Aloes, Camphor, Menthol, Peppermint, Asafoetida, Valerian, Turpentine, Carbolic Acid, etc. They should be kept in special dry and dark cupboards or special rooms where they cannot get contaminated. Again let me repeat the warning on a previous page! Low potencies only should be used by lay people, unless they are advised to do otherwise by a homœopathic physician.

CHRONIC BRONCHITIS

Can Homœopathy do anything for chronic bronchitis?

In such a variable climate as ours, the lot of the bronchial individual is not enviable. The rich bronchial patient is ordered out of England for the duration of the period of prolonged fogs and rains and cold winds by his doctor, and usually spends the months of exile in Egypt or the Canary Islands. The poorer classes have to put up with it and haunt the out-patient halls of the various hospitals, going from tuberculosis hospital or dispensary to a general hospital or infirmary or vice versa in the vain hope of getting relief. Their sputums are tested, their chests are X-rayed and, if found positive, they are drafted on to sanatoria, and rest, and good food and fresh air in an early case does often work wonders. If no tubercular germs are found, they are dubbed chronic and kept under observation, given one of the brands of Mist. Tussis co. of the hospital pharmacopæias, and fall then into the hands of the junior resident staff. They cough and spit all through the day and often through the night; even the slightest fog aggravates the condition so that it almost becomes unbearable. The slightest exertion makes them so breathless that it is painful to see them walk and crawl along the streets; the wiser, of course, stay indoors by the fire and only venture out to get a fresh supply of their favourite cough mixture from the panel doctor or hospital.

I remember such a case—a poor, under-sized, miserable specimen of humanity, first seen in June, 1931, at the age of 34, when she was four months pregnant and came for treatment for an almost complete procidentia uteri (uterine prolapse). The uterus was replaced and a medium-sized pessary was inserted to keep up the heavy pregnant uterus. She gave a history of having been "chesty" all her life since the age of three, following on an attack of measles. She had attended the local infirmary for months for suspected pulmonary tuberculosis, the periods stayed away for months as well, which pointed to early tuberculosis. Then she

was drafted to the tuberculosis dispensary and kept under observation and had repeated sputum tests and X-rays. Nothing
definite was ever found. The baby was born in due course, a
miserable infant, naturally; the prolapse recurred afterwards, and
there was some subinvolution of the uterus, the pessary was
renewed, and one lost sight of her for ten months.

In the meantime she continued to attend the tuberculosis dispensary and the nearby large teaching hospital for further tests
and X-rays of her chest. On February 9th, 1933, she came to have
her pessary changed and again she complained of irregularity of
the monthlies and wondered whether she was pregnant. The
uterus was heavy and bulky and cervix unhealthy, eroded and
inflamed. She was thin and miserable, I noticed the dirty greyish
skin, the dirty, ill-kept, untidy clothes and general lack of personal spruceness. On these general signs she was given *Sulphur* 6
night and morning for two weeks, the first time ever she had any
medicine from this department. She really came for her prolapse,
not for her general condition; in these modern days there is so
much specialization, and the patient wanders from one department to another, and in the end perhaps nobody does him or her
much good. Again she was lost sight of for five months; she only
reported in passing that her periods had been regular since
February 16th. The poor always keep a careful tally of their
monthlies, for fear of something happening.

On July 20th, 1933, she turned up again and had another
course of *Sulphur* 6, and then reported she had no bronchial
trouble since February, the time she had been given the *Sulphur*,
and indeed the tuberculosis dispensary had discharged her now.
On February 19th, 1934, a year after being first treated for her
general debility, she reported she had been slightly chesty again
during the foggy weather, and that the "periods were dodging
her," and that she had pain on top of the head. *Tuberculinum*
30, weekly doses, were given, as there had been this indefinite
history of a doubtful tubercular infection in the past. These
symptoms were really *Sulphur* symptoms, but I thought
Tuberculinum should now be given. She disappeared again
for seven months, and at the end of September, 1934, reported
that she was feeling well, and that she had no further aches on
top of the head.

Five months later (end of February, 1935) no period since

October 24th. Pains on top of the head. Eyes water and discharge. Giddy at night. Feels faint with heats. *Sulphur* 30. The period came on promptly on March 3rd, and in June, 1935, she reported that she had no further headaches; there was no asthma and no bronchitis. Her chest trouble had sometimes been called asthma and sometimes chronic bronchitis. Periods regular every month since March (the *Sulphur* was given end of February). Again a dose of *Sulphur* 30 given on this date (June 6th, 1935).

January 9th, 1936. No asthma, no bronchitis, complains of pains right leg and cramps of right leg for several weeks. The prolapse she originally came for hardly troubled her at all. Feeling well otherwise. *Sulphur* 30 again.

May 14th, 1936. Feeling very well. No chest trouble.

October 5th, 1936. Thirty-nine years old. Periods scanty again. Complains of pains bottom of back and hot sweats. *Sulphur* 30.

December 14th 1936. Very well. Prolapse hardly noticeable. Patient looks very well and feels well; no bronchitis for years. Has never been near the hospital since she was discharged in July, 1933, and she used to be an almost weekly visitor and was a sufferer from a "winter cough" since infancy.

A very satisfactory result indeed. Our books are full of records of cases of empyema, chronic bronchitis, emphysema, who were cured by doses of homœopathic remedies.

Yea, even asthma is curable by Homœopathy, though asthma cases require to keep under treatment for years sometimes; but I hope to continue this subject at some future date.

Disappointments are common in one's work, and more so if one ploughs a lonely furrow and goes against the ideas held by the herd. It is difficult to convince some people that one can do many things, and if not cure, at any rate improve an apparently incurable condition to such an extent that life is a totally different matter ever afterwards. One gets these people so far, and then somebody comes along and puts a spoke in and the improvement stops, and one has to stand by and see a nearly cured chronic patient slide back and return to the old life. Such a case came to me some three or four years ago. A typical coster woman, 34 years old, was bringing her infant along for advice, and I noticed she had an irritating, dry cough and looked thin and ill herself. On enquiry, I found that she suffered from bronchiectasis—a chronic cavity in the lung, which had come on after an interstitial pneumonia some two or three years previously. She had been an in-patient in the local infirmary, when, after thorough investigation, X-rays and so on, this condition had been diagnosed, and she was told that nothing could be done, except that she was to empty the cavity in her lungs every morning by leaning over the side of the bed to allow the accumulation of phlegm to run out by gravity. She had terrible nights, her cough would not let her sleep, and she kept her husband awake, too, by this constant irritating cough, which was worse between 3 and 5 a.m. On first getting up she would bring up quantities of fœtid, nasty, thick matter from her lungs, and all day long there would be this dry cough, which was nearly driving her husband crazy. She had lost pounds and pounds in weight, but was content to stay as she was, for nothing could be done! I tried to reason with her, and eventually she was willing to try the treatment I suggested. I found signs of old pneumonia at the base of the right lung, and on *this* sign along with chronic cough, and the general physical make-up, a thin, lean person with tendency to distension after food, I gave her *Lycopodium* 6 night and morning. I was anxious to make an impression in this case, and on looking up the symptoms at home, I thought it might be *Kali carb.* 6.

Next week I was prepared to order *Kali carb.*; but to her great surprise and my great joy she reported that the cough had been very much better, she had filled three large sputum cups the first two mornings, and since then there had been very little phlegm, and her nights were much quieter, her husband had actually slept the night through and had wondered on waking up, whether his wife was dead, as she lay so quietly. This state of affairs went on; she improved from week to week, and was kept on *Lyc.* 6, and later *Lycopodium* 12 and then *Lyc.* 30. In three months she put on a stone in weight; the sounds in the right lung cleared up; the night cough was a thing of the past, she enjoyed her food; there was very little phlegm in the morning, and I had visions of the large cavity closing up in the lungs, and I was going to send her to the radiologist for confirmation. Alas! she suddenly became pregnant again, and with the pregnancy and after the last prescription of *Lyc.* 30 she broke out in a peculiar coppery eruption all over the body and the arms: it was a smooth eruption as if somebody had painted ladders and snakes all over her; there was no scaling and only slight irritation. I was delighted, as according to the homœopathic principles, if a skin eruption shows, this is proof that elimination of the poison in the system is taking place, and the patient is well on the way to recovery, and *the best thing is to leave well alone and not to apply any external treatment.*

Unfortunately, she went to the Maternity Hospital without saying anything to me, and there they thoroughly frightened her; they advised coal-tar lotion and coal-tar ointment, to drive the skin trouble in. So for six months she was busy anointing herself with various evil-looking ointments which eventually achieved their purpose; that is healing up the skin and, of course, the cough returned as badly as ever, the foul-smelling phlegm began to run out from the lungs again and she was in *status quo.* I tried to persuade her to leave the ointment alone; but it was no use; I was the voice of one crying in the wilderness, the hospital doctor said ointment had to be applied and he had also said there was no cure for her other trouble, the chest, and the apparent preliminary improvement under the treatment was just a coincidence.

I felt like shaking the woman, but the consensus of opinion was against Homœopathy, and I heard that the husband had murmured in the background he wished she would continue with the white pills, they did seem to do her good, and he had good nights during the few months she took them!

Homœopathy had succeeded in improving this woman so far that the goal was well in sight. Another three months would have sufficed in curing the cavity completely : in fact, when she started to put the ointment on, she had no symptoms, there was neither cough nor phlegm; sound health-giving sleep, and good appetite. The drying up of the septic cavity had caused this woman to blossom forth, and then to see all this work spoilt and see her going back again to her old condition was heart breaking. One saw the woman for another two years off and on; one could always tell her presence in the dispensary by the metallic dry cough, and as she preferred the cough and the disgusting purulent phlegm to the skin eruption, which would have been a temporary and passing state of affairs, one had to leave her to it.

If only people would realize that a deep-seated condition of important internal organs can be cured and is curable; often, it is true, at the cost of temporary cosmetic discomfort; that the cure comes from within, and that the external evidence of disease should not be interfered with, except by giving the correct medicine, the medicine indicated by the symptoms, and given according to the homœopathic principles—that like cures like—that the skin is an important organ of elimination and that through the skin we throw out all kinds of effete matter; that respiration also takes place through the skin, and if we clog up all the pores of the skin by putting on a lot of grease and all sorts of ointments, we do infinite harm to such organs as the lungs, and heart and liver, where the damage does not show to the eye, it is true, but it is there nevertheless. Only very few doctors understand this; the schools have forgotten this important truth since the days of Erasmus Wilson who discovered that skin diseases could be made to disappear and were therefore pronounced cured, by external applications. Later, these skin cases developed chronic lung and heart troubles, but then they came into the province of the heart or lung specialist, and the part of the skin specialist in producing the serious internal disease was overlooked. Some time, one hopes, this sequence of events will be rediscovered, and then we shall see true "cures," cures from within outwards. This is another great homœopathic principle, that cures takes place from within outwards; serious internal disease disappears after external manifestations.

Still another more gratifying case of chronic bronchitis in a young married woman, with the following history : operation for left-sided empyema at the age of five; troublesome cough ever since then; always worse during winter, very severe during the winter of 1933. First seen in February, 1934 : had much treatment, latterly had been given Kreosote among other things : X-rayed and nothing definite found. Kept her husband awake in the early mornings by a most distressing dry cough from 2 o'clock on until 5 or 6 a.m. : irritation behind sternum, has palpitations when walking any distance, worse mornings, during cough and going up stairs : gets a cold every time she goes out. Periods are irregular all the winter, very scanty, no clots, it comes on for two days every week or every two weeks—coughs and coughs without stopping for an hour or two at a time; coughed constantly while being interrogated and being examined. Husband says "enough to drive him mad"; patient hates music, is easily irritated, feels weak all over, gets indigestion easily, feels cold very much : weight 6 stones 7 lbs. in clothes; râles and rhonchi and dullness right base of lung. Prescription *Kali carb.* 6 night and morning.

Seen again on April 19th, 1934. Period regular for two months; every month not every week as before. Never had a bad attack of coughing since her first visit in February : felt ill and seedy for the first week after taking the medicine, but quite different now, and sleeps well now. *Kali carb.* 30.

May 31st, 1934. Caught a cold two weeks ago; not sleeping so well now, coughs again between 2 to 3 a.m., loose cough with thick phlegm—weight 7 stones 6 lbs., she gained nearly a stone in three months! Periods have been regular every month. *Kali carb.* 30 nightly for a week.

September 17th, 1934. Weight 7 stones 8 lbs.; slight returns of the symptoms, palpitations, no pains in chest; caught a cold last week; on examination found again some râles behind right base of lung : the first time since February. *Dulcamara* 12 nightly for the acute condition; followed by *Kali carb.* 6.

November 28th, 1934. Very well until cold last week after a fog; loose cough which keeps her awake at night; tickling behind sternum; feels the dry cold very much *Rumex crispus* 6 t.d.s. for acute condition, and *Kali carb.* 1m. Since that time one has not seen her, but one hears through a sister that she is keeping well and has no return of cough, even though she may get colds. Her husband is very thankful, he gets peaceful nights now, he had laughingly threatened to divorce her if she did not cease her coughing.

A chronic cough of many years' duration cured by homœopathic remedies without change of air, cod-liver oil and malt and other adjuvants; the patient remaining in the same district, having the same food; nothing is altered except a little medicine is given. Carbonate of Potash or *Kali carb.* in varying potencies, which has the characteristic symptoms as given by this patient, relieved her of her troublesome complaint : her metabolism was changed for the better, and she rapidly put on weight, a stone in a few months.

Homœopathy does not let you down, if you are willing to learn about it and study it. There are many remedies which can and do cure bronchitis, whether acute or chronic; each remedy has its own particular and distinctive symptoms. The difficulty is : finding the remedy. It means constant study : willing to sit at the feet of Hahnemann and his followers, willing to learn from the knowledge which you can find in the many Materia Medica books. Start reading and studying Nash and Allen's *Keynotes*, and later Kent's *Materia Medica* and Clarke's *Dictionary of Materia Medica.*

It is a fascinating study; well worth while when you are faced with acute diseases and find you are able to cut short these acute illnesses, your pneumonias, your measles, your whooping coughs, your influenzas; that you have no fear of typhoid, of cholera, of diphtheria, of serious septic diseases; that you do not get any complications after acute diseases when you give homœopathic medicines; and the more you search, the more Homœopathy will offer you. You will be able to cure many hitherto incurable diseases and be a true healer.

ANIMAL CURES

MANY years ago, at the end of a long and tiring day, I was greeted on arriving home with the news that my little puppy had suddenly taken ill. On going to his basket I saw a distressing sight: the poor wee beastie was lying there practically unconscious, barely breathing, saliva was dribbling from his mouth, his body felt almost icy cold, even though he was bedded in a warm room; the skin was dry and harsh, the nose cold and dry, and very pale; no, or very little, pulse could be felt.

I tried to cover him up, but was assured that he had crept away from the hot bottle and had refused to remain under the blanket. What was to be done? I knew practically nothing about canine diseases; I had heard about distemper vaguely; but what the symptoms were or the treatment, I had not the foggiest notion. But I had faith in my "wee sweeties" and I said to myself: "Well, in a human being with these symptoms—sudden acute attack, great coldness, and with it aversion to being covered up, great weakness, pallor—all this meant *Camphor*"; so why not give *Camphor*?

I only had it very high, in the 2,000th potency; would it act in a dog? It was easy to give: the little sweet powder was gently put on his tongue, and very anxiously we waited for a response. In a remarkably short time he opened his eyes and feebly tried to lick my fingers, which I had dipped in warm milk and drop doses of brandy. Joyfully he was fed with a little more milk and brandy, the first nourishment he had deigned to take for hours. Next morning quite a different spectacle met me; he had crawled out of his basket, and was lying in front of the fire; gaily wagging his tail as usual in the morning.

All his coldness had disappeared, there was no more diarrhœa, there were no further signs of collapse—was it distemper? I do not know. His illness only lasted for one short night, and he recovered as quickly as he was stricken down, after taking that one dose of *Camphor*.

It had another interesting after-effect. We could not teach the little beast to be clean before. No amount of coaxing, scolding or punishment made any impression on him. But after this illness and the quick improvement he changed completely. He became quite house-clean and quite an exemplary dog.

Was that his way of showing gratitude for being made well?

"Our Tim," a beautiful tabby Persian cat, is monarch of all he surveys, and he rules the humans whom he owns with a benevolent tyranny.

A few weeks ago "Our Tim" developed a chill: the first sign of it was vomiting and some diarrhœa, which was treated with *Rhus. toxicodendron*, as he is very fond of sitting about on the cold stone steps and damp grass in the garden. It usually cuts short any feverish attacks, but this time it was of no use. The illness had gone too far and within twenty-four hours it had attacked the bladder. Very imperiously he was always demanding to be let out. The constant urging got worse and worse, and "my lord" had to use his box in the cellar. He used to look apologetically at first at his mistress, "he could not really help it." But later he was too far gone and he practically lived in his box, standing up continuously straining, just to pass a few drops.

The homœopathic Cat book recommended *Cantharis* for this trouble. However, after trying it for twenty-four hours and not noticing the slightest improvement, the *Repertory* was referred to, and the different symptoms looked up. First it was noticed that the cat, usually very fond of warmth, preferred to lie about on the cold tiles or in a cold, unheated room, away from his mistress, a most unheard of procedure, as though he had found the heat of the fire was unbearable. He did not like hot clothes on his bladder at all—a suggestion of the vet. Then there was constant straining to pass water, just a few drops; the urine was extremely concentrated and offensive.

All this pointed to *Apis*. So *Apis* was given and produced a definite aggravation for a quarter of an hour, then he settled down and went to sleep for five to six hours, curled up in a ball instead of lying stretched out straight, which he had not done since his illness began two days before. So *Apis* was repeated several times, whenever the urging frequency began to show itself, which was usually every four to five hours, and within forty-eight hours the frequency had disappeared, the offensiveness had gone. He had *Apis* for about three days and there was no need for any other medication. And the cat is now as fit and lively as ever before.

Now another case of dysuria and strangury in a cat, which occurred two or three years ago. This tom-cat was frequently attacked with pain on passing water, and used to strain and strain and nothing would pass at all. He was in acute agony and all the local vet. could suggest was warmth and hot cloths on the abdomen. He diagnosed stone in the bladder, and after two or three attacks shrugged his shoulders and suggested putting the cat to sleep. I heard about it, and, finding out that this cat was extremely fond of sitting hunched up for hours on cold stone floors in the damp weather and these attacks always came on afterwards, I prescribed *Rhus. Toxicodendron* in the 6th centesimal potency, which acted promptly, and since that time his mistress always keeps *Rhus. tox.* in the house and, at the slightest sign of bladder trouble, he gets a dose and nothing further happens to distress him. The fame of this prescription spread over to Paris, where an American friend, who is a cat lover, had one of her cats attacked with this agonizing trouble and whose vet. also advised getting rid of her pet. She gave him some *Rhus. tox.* and lo, and behold! it cleared up at once.

Now for a story about a dog :

He was only a little black mongrel in a little slum street, beloved play companion of some little friends of mine. He always used to greet me with such a jolly bark, such hearty tail-wagging, when I arrived. One morning I missed his exuberant welcome. "Where is 'Pat'?" I enquired, after I had finished with my little measles patients. "Oh! he has bronchitis and is not well," the mother told me and, on going to his kennel, this was the picture that greeted me. My dog friend was curled up in his kennel which was lined with blankets and rugs. "He was so cold," apologized his mistress, "I had to put an extra rug over him." The door of his kennel was fastened and hung over with a blanket. "Why did you fasten the door?" I asked. "Oh, he is so badtempered, so unlike himself, he threatened to bite us." And when I went up to him he rose up shivering and trembling with cold and growled at me and showed his teeth, a most unusual behaviour in this friendly little dog, and the breathing was very rapid. I could not examine him, as he was so bad-tempered and unapproachable; but I left some *Nux vomica* powder with his mistress with full instructions. Two days later when I saw him, he was his old friendly self again, all signs of bronchitis had disappeared. Another triumph for Homœopathy!

Were these cures really faith cures, as enemies of Homœopathy declare? Faith may move mountains, but faith alone on my part did not cure "Our Tim" when *Cantharis* was given for his cystitis. It required the properly indicated drug, the drug which, according to homœopathic law, was the right drug, before any impression was made on the disease. The same with the bronchitis in the dog. *Nux vomica* does not cure every case of bronchitis in a dog. It only cured this dog's bronchitis as the symptoms, the extreme coldness, the extreme irritability—even turning against his dear mistress and biting her—pointed to *Nux vomica*. So in human beings. A remedy chosen according to the Law will cure, and cure rapidly, provided it is the right remedy.

To be owned by a cat is almost as responsible a job as being owned and tyrannized over by a child: and cats, moreover, are very difficult beings to treat when they are ill as they don't tell you anything, and are so passive, so lacking in spunk that they just as lief die as make a fight for it, as dogs invariably do. You have to watch the feline tribe very carefully, both in health and disease, or they quietly slip out of your life without much ado. I expect it is because they are secretive and always like to walk by themselves, that they manage to be almost dead before you have realized that they are ill. We had many alarums and excursions with "Our Tim"—one of the nearest shaves we had was last winter, when being in the throes of a domestic upheaval, and the latest one being a particularly unpleasant type of the "femina domestica" who neglected and drove the poor cat out of doors in the worst kinds of weather. Nobody had been told of his refusal to touch his food until it was palpable even to the lay mind that something very serious was up: Tim refused to stir from his armchair; for days he just lay drowsily stretched out, would not touch any tit-bits that were offered him. He passed by the daintiest morsels of best English steak and liver which he could never resist, as a rule. He turned his nose up at rich creamy milk and only wished to be left alone. All the normal body functions seemed to be at a standstill, and he rapidly wasted away in a few days until he was but skin and bones, and so weak he could barely open his eyes or open his mouth and swallow his food. He had to be forcibly fed twice a day by hand. Two ounces of raw meat were cut up fine and pushed far back down his throat, or he would just let it slide out of his mouth again. He was also spoonfed with warm milk with a dash of brandy in it.

There were very few symptoms except this utter laziness, this refusal to stir, this absolute do-nothing attitude and a refusal to be kept warm, though he is naturally a beast who adores the warmest place. On these few symptoms he was given *Sulphur* 30 night and morning and then *Sulphur m.* daily for nearly a fortnight. When he was at his worst he weighed less than 7 lbs., the normal weight being 10¼ lbs. After a fortnight of anxiety he decided it was no good resisting any more and he started to eat again, and once he liked the taste of food again he became so ravenous that he soon more than made up his loss of weight. One saw in the papers that at that time there was a general epidemic of cat influenza in the neighbourhood and practically 100 per cent. died; so once again Homœopathy and careful nursing and hand feeding saved a life, even though it might be only that of a dumb animal.

Some time afterwards we had another alarum. The poor beast had to be sent to a vet.'s to be boarded while his mistress went on a long-needed holiday. He came back somewhat jaded and rather worse for wear, having lost half a pound in weight. Worse was to follow: one day soon after his return, a large bald patch was noticed on his back, a round circular patch; by this time the size of a five-shilling piece—and there was the ominous red scaly line on the circumference. Alas! it was nothing else but the dreaded ringworm of the hair. What to do, was the question. Send him back to the vet., or treat him at home? It was decided to give Homœopathy a chance again, and on studying Jahr's *Forty Years' Practice*, a very valuable old homœopathic book full of the most useful practical hints, we found this suggestion of painting a ringworm patch with oil of lavender and apply the indicated remedy as well.

Unfortunately we found the ringworm had spread a good deal further besides the large bare patch, but, nothing daunted, the treatment was begun. The remedy chosen was the favourite one of the late Dr. Burnett's for ringworm, namely *Bacillinum* 30, which was given twice a week at first and then once weekly. He responded very nicely, for which thanks be to old Jahr and Burnett for their pearls of wisdom.

The further spread of the skin disease was arrested at once, but it took about six weeks before the hair completely covered the bald patch. Baldness of the scalp due to X-ray treatment after ringworm takes six months before the hair covers the whole of the scalp again. This reminds me of a case of ringworm of the scalp in a child of seven years which one saw more than a decade ago. It had been treated scientifically for months without any sign of a cure : the hair was all off and yet the parasite was still there, so active indeed, that the writer became infected and developed ringworm of the neck within a few days. This child was given *Bacillinum* 30 and later *Bacillinum m.*, and within a week of the first dose his hair started to sprout and the scales disappeared, and no further sign of the parasite was found, microscopically.

But *revenons à nos moutons*, or rather to our cats. As you have seen, Homœopathy acts rapidly in cats. You only need to watch them carefully and then choose the indicated remedy. Skin diseases in cats are common enough, alas! they are such rovers and you cannot keep them away, as in the case of dogs, from other members of their tribe.

There was a beautiful black Persian cat I knew who developed mange, her whole trunk was covered. The vet. advised its destruction. Do they ever advise anything else for cats if there is anything serious the matter with pussy? The owner of the Persian was willing to try Homœopathy and *Sulphur* 6 was given faithfully night and morning for several weeks, followed by complete recovery.

One came across another cat in one's wanderings, a very old tabby, who had developed a nasty growth from his ear in the shape of a black curved horn, about two inches long. He was given *Thuja* 30, daily doses for a week, and the horn promptly fell off and had not recurred again six months later. One wishes that there were homœopathic vets. so that our pets could be saved instead of being destroyed prematurely.

THE COMMON COLD AND ITS TREATMENT

THE common cold is a disgrace and constant reproach to the medical profession. So far it has beaten all the efforts of the doctors to conquer it. In common cold I include all varieties from a mild nasal catarrh to a more or less serious systemic reaction with pyrexia and general malaise, a rise of temperature and a feeling of being sick. The usual instructions of isolation at the first signs of a cold, by staying in bed for a couple of days on a light diet is good as far as it goes, it prevents the general spread of infection, but it is just a remnant of the "leave it to nature and do nothing else school" and certainly better than the recent more drastic fads of the bug-hunting, serum-injecting apostles of the Pasteur school who are a positive danger to the health of the future generation. No, there are safer, more expeditious means of fighting and conquering the ubiquitous cold than the various broths concocted in the kitchens of the modern alchemists who are looking for the elixir of life among the by-products of the transmutation of healthy cells, the various degenerating forms of bacteria, cocci, moulds and the rest.

The first line of defence should be the injunction, keep yourself fit by all the means at your command, doing graduated exercises daily in the open air, not just violent exercise once a week, leading an open-air life whenever possible promoting the action of the skin by open-air baths clad in the minimum of clothes. But do not make the mistake of becoming a nuisance to your fellow creatures by selfishly insisting on opening all the windows in a bus or railway carriage in a cold wind or thick fog, for gradually becoming chilled by sitting still for hours in a cool or draughty atmosphere often leads to neuralgia, colds and even pneumonia. It is sufficient to open the window in a compartment for a couple of minutes every half-hour for purposes of ventilation. Do not spend too much time in crowded, ill-ventilated halls or rooms, cinemas, theatres and dance halls during the season when colds are prevalent. Eat and drink in moderation, do not partake too freely of starchy foods, go slow on meat, take as much cleansing alkaline food as you can such as fresh fruit when available, add raw vegetable salads to your meals, drink vegetable juices daily such as spinach water, cabbage water, etc. A starchy diet of buns, cakes and pastries plus tinned meats, meat pies, and sausages produces acidity of the blood which is a favourable breeding ground for a variety of diseases. The next defence line is the positive therapy of the homœpathic medication. Therefore keep under a homœpathic physician who by constitutional treatment throughout the year will raise the resistance to colds and other acute infections. The last defence line for an acute cold is the prescription of the correct remedy for each attack.

Now there is no specific remedy for a cold. It depends on a variety of circumstances which particular remedy will cure your special brand of cold each time, and the remedy which cured your cold last go, may fail utterly at the next attack, therefore consider first and foremost what are the circumstances which determine the remedy for different types of colds. First of all it depends on the meteorological conditions or, in other words, on the weather prevailing on the day you caught the cold. Now follows a list of remedies which are of value in fighting different kinds of colds.

Chill or coryza after exposure to a draught: Aconite, Calcarea, Ferr, Hepar., Merc.

Exposure to draught when heated: Aconite, Carbo. veg., Silica.

Exposure to draught when perspiring: Bryonia.

Exposure to rain: Ars., Bell., Calc., Dulc., Ferr., Nat. sulph., Rhus. tox.

Sleeping in damp rooms or beds: Ars., Calc., Carbo. veg., Nat. sulph., Rhus. tox.

Staying at seaside: Nat. mur., Nat. sulph.

Standing in water: Rhus. tox.

From becoming wet: Acon., Bell., Bry., Calc., Nat. sulph., Rhus tox.

From wet feet: Merc., Nat. carb., Nat. mur., Phos., Puls., Rhus., tox., Sep., Sil.

Becoming wet when overheated: Acon., Calc., Rhus. tox.

Sudden chill from bathing in cold water when hot or having a cold shower when getting hot at games: Bellis-perennis.

Working in clay or in water: Calc., Rhus. tox.

Cold damp wind: Allium cepa.

Hot weather of summer : Bapt., Bell., Bry.

Chill in Spring : Ars., Carbo. veg., Gels., Lach., Psor., Sep., Sulph.

Autumnal colds : Ars., Bapt., Bry., Nat. mur., Nux. vom., Rhus. tox., Sepia.

Autumn and Spring : Ars., Lach., Psor., Sep.

Caused by anxiety : Acute stage Aconite (developing suddenly on the same day); Ars., Gels. (in mild relaxing weather); Tuberc. for recurring colds.

After excitement : Calc., Gels. Ignatia.

From fright : Acon., Ars., Bry., Gels., Ign., Lyc., Merc., Nux. vom., Op., Puls., Sil.

From grief : Gels., Ign.

After vexation : Acon., Ars., Bry., Gels., Merc., Nux. vom., Rhus. tox.

After exposure to cold dry weather and cold winds : Acon. (same day), Asarum (in thin neurotic persons), Causticum, Hepar, Kali carb., Nux. vom. (all two to three days after exposure).

Snowy weather : Puls., Rhus. tox.

Cloudy weather : Bry., Cham., Chin., Dulc., Puls., Rhux. tox. and Sulph.

Cold damp weather : Ars., Calc., Dulc., Rhus. tox., Sulph.

The psychological effects of emotions produce a lowering effect on the constitution and resistance to chills. The commonly accepted notion is that colds are caught from other people; but what about the individual who starts the ball rolling? And what explanation is there for the people who are always taking colds, and their neighbours who remain free from colds? The unknown factor x is, of course, the individual himself and the state of health he is in.

Having decided that a particular cold is due to certain prevailing weather conditions, you have to find out which of these half a dozen or more weather remedies is the most similar to the type of cold to be cured. Some people always run to *Aconite* as soon as a cold or feverish chill develops and in England colds are very rarely *Aconite* colds. *Aconite* is a chill coming on after cold dry winds, it shows itself first in the evening, the patient is restless, anxious, fearful, with a very red flushed face, tossing about with agony, skin is dry and hot without any sweat and the fear is usually the fear of dying without any signs of delirium. If these symptoms are present a feverish chill will be cured in a few hours with Aconite.

A more common remedy in England for early stages of colds is *Arsenic. Arsenic* is always taking cold, suffers from draughts, worse cold, damp weather, sneezing from every change in the weather, cold begins in the nose and goes down into the throat and then to the chest; a hard dry tickling cough, thirst for sips of warm water which relieve; is restless, weak and prostrated.

Baptisia is an acute, rapidly acting medicine, the patient is attacked suddenly, is prostrated, stupid, is restless, tosses about, confused as if intoxicated, wakes up anxious and startled from sleep; in his delirium thinks there are two or more of him; it is a toxic case, an intensified *Gels.* condition, which see later for comparison. Remember the restlessness is different from the *Arsenic* restlessness, there is less fear and more delirium in *Baptisia.*

Belladonna cold and chill comes on after a haircut or the hair being washed; exposure to cold winds, in chubby children and vigorous, plethoric adults. The chill comes on with great suddenness, runs a rapid course and subsides as suddenly, is associated with violent heat, brilliant red face and throat, intense redness, intense burning and throbbing; there is no fear as in *Aconite*, there is delirium instead, fear of imaginary things, violent delirium.

Some people like to alternate *Aconite* and *Belladonna*, this should never be necessary, as they are totally different in their action. *Bryonia* is frequently indicated in this damp, maritime climate of ours, cold comes on after every change in the weather. It comes on gradually, takes several days to develop, the patient feels mouldy, gradually feeling worse; so different from *Aconite, Belladonna* and *Baptisia*, which come on suddenly. The *Bry.* chill starts with sneezing, running of the nose, aching through eyes and head, gradually it goes down into the throat, bronchitis and even pneumonia may follow; there is great thirst in feverish conditions for cold water, large quantities of water at long intervals. The patient looks stupid, sleeps a lot, is confused, the face is congested, mottled and purple, he does not want to move as motion makes all the pains worse, coughing is painful, has to press his hands against his chest and abdomen when he coughs; remember always that *Bryonia* is worse from movement, is better for pressure.

Gelsemium colds and chills come on slowly and gradually; take several days to develop, come on after getting over-heated in warm, mild winters or chills in summer; often caused by emotional upsets, fear, grief, nerves, anticipation of trouble; the face is congested, mottled, purple, cold shivers running up the spine to the back of the head, sneezing with hot face and red eyes, lies still, does not want to stir or move, because of the heaviness and the weight of the limbs and body, wants to be left alone, does not want to talk; there is no thirst, hot face with coldness of the extremities. *Gels.* is not so toxic as *Baptisia*, not so intensely red or violently delirious as *Belladonna*. *Hepar sulph.* is likely to get a nasal cold or croup every time he goes out in a cold north-east wind. Loss of voice and a dry, barking cough with hoarseness, cough is worse when putting hands and feet out of the bed; or there may be much sneezing with a running of a clear watery discharge which ends up by becoming thick, yellow and offensive; the cold develops slowly within twenty-four hours after exposure. *Aconite* is usually the first prescription, if it does not hold, *Spongia* comes next, and then *Hepar*.

Allium Cepa comes on after exposure to a biting, cold damp wind, west, south-west or north-west winds in England, and is specific remedy for colds with its own peculiar symptoms. I knew an old lady, an aristocrat to her fingertips, well on in the eighties, who was a great believer in *Allium Cepa* for colds. She used to dispense it freely among her friends in her walks abroad, the stall-holders in the street markets, the flower-sellers of Hyde Park and Marble Arch, the crossing-sweepers, policemen and postmen, and she swore she cured them very quickly of their colds and coughs. Of course she was quite right, for they were all workers sitting or standing at draughty street corners, exposed to the vagaries of the weather, the cold damp westerly winds whistling down the streets and round the old squares. People standing in queues waiting for buses may often develop *Allium cepa* colds. The nose becomes raw, especially on the left side, the watery discharge is copious and produces sores on nose and lips from the constant drip, profuse flow of water from the left eye which is painless and bland, later the throat and larynx get inflamed and raw, there is a tearing pain in the larynx with each cough. The patient is hot and thirsty, the cold is worse in the evenings and indoors like *Puls*.

Mercurius, repeated catarrhs during winter in people who are constantly taking cold, which it cures at once, but if *Merc.* is taken too often it makes the patient more sensitive to colds, it should not therefore be taken more than twice during the winter, a deeper acting constitutional remedy must be taken instead of *Merc.* The symptoms are a burning in the face, a running cold, profuse watery discharge, peculiar creeping chilliness followed by profuse sweating which does not relieve the catarrh; worse from the warmth of the bed. The *Merc.* cold starts in the head and travels down the throat and larynx to the bronchial tubes.

Nux vomica, gets a cold every time he is bilious and whenever his digestion goes wrong. These people should attend to their diet, eschew all rich food and live only on the simplest, avoid coffee, wine and cocktails and then the tendency to colds would disappear. Unfortunately their stomach is their god and you cannot often persuade them to give up the pleasure of the table; *Nux vom.* gets a chill after exposure to the dry east and north-east winds, the slightest current of air causes a catarrh which is worse in a stuffy, heated room, the nose is stuffed up at night in the house, but runs freely if out of doors, splitting headache, great soreness of chest, feels extremely chilly, has to sit crouched over the fire and has to pile on extra bedclothes, shivers on the slightest movement in bed, is extremely irritable and snappy with it.

Pulsatilla, subject to frequent colds with sneezing and stuffing up of the nose in the morning with thick, yellow-green discharge; in the evening there is much watery discharge with sneezing, pains in the face and through the nose, worse indoors and better out of doors, clear thick mucus collects in the throat, loss of smell and taste is often present; there is no thirst, even if the temperature is high.

Rhus tox. chills come on after getting soaked or wet, living in a damp house or sleeping in a damp bed, pains in the eyes, the nose is stopped up, the tongue is sore and raw and red, the thirst is violent, glands of the neck are swollen and the neck is stiff. The cold may extend into the larynx with hoarseness, a dry teasing cough, great restlessness; all symptoms are worse on first moving about.

Camphor in a low potency is prescribed routinely by some doctors in the early stages of a cold, on the indication of great coldness of the external surface of the body and sensation of cold wind blowing on it, in repeated doses half-hourly. It may abort a cold if given just as soon as the first indication appears; from personal experience I have found other drugs such as *Arsenic, Bryonia, Nux Vomica* or *Pulsatilla* of much greater use, given according to the symptoms found in the early stages.

Natrum mur., the salt remedy, works very well in certain colds, especially where there is a tendency to cold sores, herpes on the upper lip and in those people who are always worse at the seaside. It removes the tendency to colds; patients who are extremely sensitive to changes in the weather, worse from change of cold to warm; the catarrhal discharge is like the white of an egg, the patient is chilly in the mornings round about ten o'clock and takes cold easily after sweating. The constitutional *Nat. mur.* symptoms must be present such as weeping when annoyed, worse consolation, brooding over unpleasant occurrences, worse both extremes of heat and cold, craving for salt and a loathing of fat.

Kali bichromicum is affected by exposure to damp cold, worse from the melting of the snow. The nasal discharge is copious, thick yellow, almost too sticky to blow out, accompanied by much pain at the root of the nose to the outer angle of the eye.

Such constitutional remedies as sulphur, calcarea, psorinum, tuberculinum may be necessary to break up a series of repeated colds, the choice must be made on the symptoms found in the particular patient.

Just an example of the rapidity of the action of the correctly indicated remedy. A refugee student at a residential home for children was seen on a Friday morning in the autumn of 1938 suffering from a feverish chill with a stuffy nose, dry mouth and slightly inflamed throat, temperature only 99.4°. History of repeated streptococcal throats was given. Aspirin had already been given four-hourly by the orthodox matron; hot lemon drinks and barley water were prescribed plus a tepid compress round the neck with saline gargles. As it appeared to be only a mild infection the four-hourly medication of Aspirin was not interfered with, I was somewhat curious as to what would happen if the aspirin would really stop the infection; the next morning the girl was very much worse, the temperature which had gone up to nearly 104° the previous evening was still 103° at 9 a.m., she was drowsy, listless and thirstless in spite of her high temperature and had passed a sleepless night; the throat was very inflamed and congested, a typically septic throat; *Pulsatilla* 30 in watery solution to be taken two-hourly was ordered; that evening the temperature went down to 99°, on Sunday morning the temperature was normal, the throat had cleared up, the patient was hungry, mentally alert after a good night, had ordinary meals that day and wanted to get up. Because of the previous history of septic throats she was kept in bed another two days and sent away to friends in the country for the rest of the week. There was no recurrence of the septic throat during the whole of that winter. The girl herself as well as the matron were extremely astonished at the rapidity of the cure and feeling of well-being while the medicine was acting. This quick recovery made quite a stir in that community and Homœopathy became well established there as a result.

Colds and feverish chills can be cured rapidly in the home by our remedies and much serious ill-health can be avoided in consequence, if lay people would familiarise themselves with these drugs, a few of which have been mentioned in detail in this chapter, but do not change the medicine too frequently, observe the symptoms carefully and compare them with the symptoms of the drugs and, after having found the drug which is most like the variety of cold present, dissolve it in half a tumbler of water, take a teaspoonful every two hours until improvement sets in, then lengthen the intervals to four hours and stop when the cold has cleared up. If there is no improvement in 24 hours, or there is a change in the character of the chill by the next day, look up your remedies again and prescribe accordingly. Therefore the right way of treating a cold is: observe the patient, know your remedies properly, and then good luck to you, you will be successful and gain a reputation for curing colds in your own immediate circle of friends.

MORE ABOUT POTENCIES

AT a discussion the other day I found that the question of potencies and of potentisation was not clearly understood and was a constant source of mystification to the enquiring minds of people of ordinary intelligence.

When drugs were first tested, each one singly on a group of healthy subjects—mainly doctors in Hahnemann's day—it was found that each drug produced a certain number of reactions or symptoms, peculiarly belonging to that drug or medicinal substance; and no other drug, however similar it appeared to the superficial observer, yielded the same number or variety of symptoms, that is, they were specific for that particular drug.

Let us take the analogy of a white man going to an island in the Antipodes. At first, all the islanders look alike to him; but after a shorter or longer stay, according to his powers of observation, he begins to notice differences in the shape of the features, the nose, the ear, the mouth and the gait, until at long last, he perceives that each one is an individual and different from all the rest. It is the same with the hundreds of drugs which have been proved, worked out and a scheme drawn up; all by experiments on healthy men and women, the differences and the similarities between the drugs have been compared and contrasted, so that they are individualised drugs, suitable for sick persons who, when seized with an illness, which is a departure from the normal, present certain definite symptoms and reactions which vary according to the individual attacked. In other words, you treat, not the pneumonia of Mr. or Mrs. Smith, but Mr. or Mrs. Smith who has pneumonia; a vast difference.

The orthodox school of physicians on the other hand does not recognise these particular vital reactions of the different drugs; they only recognise and make use of the chemical, mechanical and physiological actions of each and every drug. For example : too much hydrochloric acid is present in the stomach, therefore the chemical antidote must be given in the shape of an alkaline remedy. The bowels do not act; stubborn and hard fæces are found, then liquid paraffin is prescribed for its mechanical action in softening the fæces. Or the uterus is bleeding, a remedy is given which physiologically produces a constriction of the dilated blood vessels of the organ as well as contraction of the musculature; Ergot does this in physiological doses and therefore it is prescribed for its physiological action in all uterine hæmorrhages.

The most vital action of medicinal substances or drugs has not been recognised by the medical school; that is, the dynamic action which is brought out by the process of potentisation which means, making more powerful or giving power. Hahnemann, by proving all his remedies on healthy individuals, found out the living and vital reactions. When he examined people with acute diseases, who each presented definite symptoms belonging to the particular person attacked by a certain disease, he compared the sick person crying out to be cured and the drug which had the power to cure, as shown by the symptoms it produced in the healthy person. When he recognised the drug similar to the disease before him, he gave that similar or most similar drug at first in material doses, drop doses as a rule. He found very soon that there followed with the similar drug a period of greater or smaller worsening of the symptoms; the negative phase of the modern pathologist. In order to reduce this negative phase, this preliminary worsening or aggravation of the disease, he began to decrease each dose. Being a scientist trained in exact methods as a mathematician and an analytical chemist, he did it, as I have already explained, according to mathematical principles by subdividing each dose on the 1 in 100 scale, and thoroughly vibrating or shaking or stirring up the drug and the diluent used at each step. He went on experimenting by dividing and subdividing each drug on the 1 in 100 scale and discovered the more he divided the dose, the more powerful became the action of the drug.

He found in fact that the lesser became the greater. A vital and most important truth. He discovered thus the dynamis, the transcendental action of each drug. "Can this be possible?" you say. To the man steeped in materialism, this seems foolish to say the least; the lesser cannot be the greater. And yet this same man, this same doctor who laughs at the possibility of being able to cure with doses of one millionth of a grain, or even a smaller quantity, this doctor shakes in his shoes at the thought of smallpox and passes on his fears to all the rest of credulous mankind.

At the mere breath of the word smallpox, all rush off to be vaccinated as a preventive, even though smallpox may be miles away at the other end of the county. And the causative agent of smallpox is a virus, an agent so small that even the strongest lenses of the most powerful microscope cannot make it visible; it is an invisible ultramicroscopic organic cell. Do you understand what that means? A bacillus which shows up moderately plainly in a microscope, is so small that it would take 400 millions of bacilli, lying side by side, to cover an ordinary postage stamp. And a virus is infinitely smaller than one bacillus. The doctors are afraid of smallpox and so is every sensible person, and with reason; for a severe case of smallpox is a truly awful spectacle and extremely fatal as well. And is not everybody scared of diphtheria, of the minute bacillus causing this disease, so deadly to so many children, which is prevalent everywhere; all the health officials rush about and are so busy getting everybody protected against it, they do not laugh or sneer at the minuteness of this organism; they have felt the power of these minute germs. Yes, they are all disease-minded, they fear diseases and their causes, the minutest cells. But they do not follow up this argument to its logical conclusion; if the infinitesimal organism has so much power for evil, why cannot an infinitesimal quantity of a drug have as much power for good?

There are all kinds of viruses, viruses causing diseases in humans, measles, mumps and smallpox, etc., there are viruses causing diseases in animals and others causing diseases in plants. We do not know how they act, but we are content to accept the fact that they do act and cause serious harm. And these same people who acknowledge the power inherent in these minutest of living forms, the viruses, will not recognise the radio-active power, the dynamic forces residing in and brought about by the special method of preparation of the potentised drugs. We know much more about them than we know about viruses. We know how the potencies are made; we know the action of each drug; they have been proved, and it has been shown, that they are able to produce definite reactions, and they have been proved not only in health but in diseases as well; the similar potentised drug by the forces freed by the special preparation by trituration or succussion according to definite mathematical rules, cures the patient with the similar disease completely and rapidly and easily. The large dose, the material dose of a drug only acts in three dimensions, but the vitally prepared, the dynamised drug, acts in the fourth dimension, and because it is smaller, certain forces previously chained inside the cell have been freed and these vibrations, millions and millions of them, have been set free by potentisation and have become the greatest power for good in the world of disease and ill-health.

The lesser in quantity has become the greater in quality.

The simillimum drug, the drug most like the disease which asks to be cured at the moment the doctor sees it, has acted for years like that, acts now and will act in the same way as long as this earth stands, for it is a law of nature, not a fiction of the brain, is not ephemeral, unless this law is forgotten and spurned by materialistic doctors.

In a certain philosophical school of medicine which flourished in a sane pre-Hitlerite Germany, a number of investigators probed into this question of the power of the minute; they made hundreds of experiments with small, smaller, and smallest doses of metals on growing plants and proved the truth of all I have said just now. They proved that comparatively large, materially large doses of metals killed the plant or plants, or strongly inhibited their growth; smaller or medium doses were more or less indifferent to the plants while the minute and minutest doses of the metals would stimulate the growth and the smaller the dose the more the growth was stimulated. Some metals would stimulate the growth of leaves, others the growth of the flowers and others would stimulate and encourage the formation of the fruit and seeds. Always it was the smallest which were most active in stimulating the plant to do its best.

Thus the truth of the Hahnemannian assertion that it is a principle of nature that small doses stimulate, while large doses kill or inhibit, was proved to be correct by these experiments on plants. Unfortunately, these telling experiments, these important investigations, have not been published yet; one only hopes they will be published some time in the near future.

The lesser in size and quantity has once again been proved to be the greater in quality and power.

I grant you, these potencies are mystifying, bewildering to minds which usually deal with sizeable things, things they can see, feel and touch. A finite mind cannot understand the mere mathematical fraction of a potentised drug. For example: the 6th potency, usually written down simply by the numeral 6, or sometimes 6*c*, means mathematically 1 over 12 noughts, or 1 over 6 double noughts, or 100^6, as the older arithmetical books show it. The 12th potency means, mathematically written, 1 over 12 double noughts, and is prepared in twelve different stages, each stage being made from the preceding one by diluting one drop in a hundred drops and shaking or succussing violently at each step. The 30th potency means 1 over 30 double noughts, a figure a finite mind cannot take in and yet, when you are a physician dealing with sick people, you find in practice, in chronic diseases you will need all potencies, that the third centesimal potency will work for a certain time, then it will cease to act; then you give the 6th potency, it will take hold of the same patient and take him along the road to health. After a time the 6th potency may fail and you will try a higher one, and once again he improves; then the patient sticks once more; you go a step higher, you go up to the 30th potency say, and again there is a steady improvement; for a time you go on giving the 30th potency and then it fails to act. If the patient still presents the same symptoms, always compare the symptoms of the patient with the symptoms of the drug at each stage, then go higher again and give the 200th potency. And so on, you gradually increase the potency, that is, lessen the quantity of the drug; but increase the radio-active vibrations; the quality of the drug and the patient will improve more and more at each raising of the potency. And so in chronic diseases, you may have to go up and up the ladder, until the desired goal is reached : that is, health. If you had started with a high potency, you would have set up such violent reactions, for the vibrations would have been too numerous and so powerful as to cause such a violent dynamic shock as to almost annihilate the patient, while if you begin low and go up step by step, you get no violent shocks, no violent reactions, just an agreeable cure. High potencies are dangerous things and as such ought to be treated with great respect.

If you know anything about astronomy, you will more easily understand and grasp the transcendental nature of a high potency. For the knowledge of the stars, the course of the stars is based on the most abstruse science of mathematical calculations. The light of the star you see at night, twinkling in the night sky, has taken sometimes thousands of years travelling through space before the light reaches your vision. It is unbelievable but true.

The astronomer can prove all kinds of abstruse mathematical

problems to you, the homœopathic physician is in advance of the necessary scientific instruments which may prove his case, that the smaller the drugs the greater is their power. But the proofs of his contention that the law of similars is correct, that the law of potentisation is correct, are coming along, and sooner or later everyone will know and have to acknowledge the correctness of this statement that the lesser is the greater in medicine.

I leave you to it now. I have tried to explain by precept and by many examples how Homœopathy works out in practice, and what Homœopathy is: namely, an individualist medicine, a therapy, a treatment by medicines taken from the three kingdoms: animal, vegetable and mineral; treating the totality of the person concerned, that is treating the physical body through the etheric body and by means of the higher potencies reaching out to the astral body and even going as far as the Ego principle, the Higher Self; and thus gradually, stage by stage, a true Healer, who is led by intuition, can touch and eradicate Karmic Sin; through prayer and fasting, with the co-operation and the true desire of the patient, all the devils can be cast out. A high ideal which is difficult to achieve.

A psychologist needs time to study his patients individually, their reactions and response to multiple tests. This is well known and acknowledged to be necessary. A homœopathic physician is a psychologist, nay, even a psychiatrist, for he studies not only the coarse reactions of a patient to his surroundings, but also traces the vagaries of the character, the aversions, the hates and the loves and the desires, and surely he must be given the right and opportunity to heal and cure his patient by the remedy which shows and has produced similar changes and reactions on the healthy person on whom it was first tested out. That is Homœopathy, individual, spiritualised vibrational medicine.

MEDICAL REFERENCES

ALLEN, H. C., Dr., *Keynotes of Leading Remedies*, 182, 190.
ALLEN, H. C., Dr., *Materia Medica*, 56.
BARKER, J. ELLIS, *Miracles of Healing*, 81.
BELL, JAMES B., Dr., *Diarrhœa and Dysentery*, 108.
BOENNINGHAUSEN, FRANZ VON, 142.
BOYD, W. E., Dr., 10.
BURDON, SANDERSON, PROFESSOR, 165.
BURFORD, G., Dr., 166–7.
BURNETT, J. C., Dr., 17, 70, 84, 96, 98–9, 101, 166, 196.
CARLETON, EDMUND, Dr., *Homœopathy in Medicine and Surgery*, 101, 148, 164.
CLARKE, JOHN H., Dr., 46, 138, 142, 156–8, 190.
DUNHAM, CAROL, Dr., 142.
DRYSDALE, Dr., 165.
ECLECTIC SCHOOL, 92.
FARRINGDON, PROFESSOR, 142.
FRANZ, Dr., 147.
GUERNSEY, E., Dr., 29.
HAHNEMANN, *Organon*, 15.

HERING, Dr., *Potentization*, 8.
HOYLE, PETRIE, Dr., 147.
HUNT, Dr., 166.
JAHR, G. H. G., *Forty Years Practice*, 196.
KENT, JAMES TYLER, Dr., *Materia Medica*, 190.
KENT, JAMES TYLER, Dr., *Repertory*, 34, 50, 117, 138, 142, 173–5, 179, 182.
LANGDON BROWN, 10.
LISTER, 81.
NASH, E. B., Dr., *Leaders in Homœopathic Therapeutics*, 182, 190.
OSLER, PROFESSOR, *Principles and Practice of Medicine*, 17–18.
PASTEUR, 81, 198.
PULFORD, A. & T., Drs., *Homœopathic Leaders in Pneumonia*, 18.
RIDPATH, Dr., 83.
SIMMELWEISS — OF VIENNA, 81.
SHERBINO, Dr., 165–6.
SHULDHAM, Dr., 166.
SIMPSON, Dr., 81.
SWAN, Dr., 165–6.
WILKINSON, D. GARTH, Dr., 96.

INDEX